3 Fat Chicks on a Diet

Produced by The Philip Lief Group, Inc.

ST. MARTIN'S GRIFFIN ❧ NEW YORK

3 Fat Chicks on a Diet

How Three Ordinary Women Battle the Bulge—and How You Can Too!

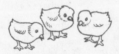

Suzanne,

Jennifer, and

Amy Barnett

with Bev West

Produced by The Philip Lief Group, Inc.

www.stmartins.com

Library of Congress Cataloging-in-Publication Data

Barnett, Suzanne.
    3 fat chicks on a diet : how three ordinary women battle the bulge—and how you can too! / Suzanne Barnett, Jennifer Barnett, and Amy Barnett; with Bev West.
        p. cm.
    ISBN-13: 978-0-312-34808-3
    ISBN-10: 0-312-34808-8
    1. Reducing diets. 2. Weight loss. 3. Dieters—Biography. I. Barnett, Jennifer. II. Barnett, Amy. III. Title.

RM222.2.B384 2006
613.2'5—dc22

                            2005033026

First St. Martin's Griffin Edition: April 2008

10 9 8 7 6 5 4 3 2 1

This book is dedicated to the wonderful, supportive members of the 3FC on-line community. Thanks to them, this book blossomed instead of our thighs.

acknowledgments

3 *FAT CHICKS ON A DIET* is the collective work of a lifetime of dieting. Many people gave us knowledge, inspiration, and support throughout our personal journeys and challenges of weight loss and the writing of this book.

Thank you, Mom and Dad, for always supporting us and encouraging us to stick with it. You've always loved us, fit or fat, and we are blessed to have you as our parents. We would also like to thank our brother, Doug Barnett, and his wife, Becky, for putting up with all the diet talk at the dinner table for all these years and for boldly trying any weird recipe that we showed up with. If anything, a few of them were a just return for the dirt and dog biscuits Doug tricked us into eating as little girls!

Suzanne would like to thank her son, Nicholas Barnett, for always encouraging her to be healthy and take care of herself, and for hiding the Little Debbie cakes from her while growing up. She'd also like to thank him for his love and support, and for taking care of things while she was holed away in the Batcave writing this book. No mother could be luckier than to have a son like you.

Jennifer would like to thank her husband, Rob Lesman, and son, Cody Honeycutt, for incredible patience and understanding while she was writing the book. Cody, you've been a sweetheart night after night while Mom worked, always being the funny guy just when it was needed. Rob, you've been Jennifer's rock through this process with your creative help and never-ending encouragement, and you've kept Jennifer's life in motion for the past year. There is no way she could have done this without you, and she is lucky to have you for a partner.

Amy would like to thank her husband, Jack Buchanan, for his support through the years, and for loving her regardless of her weight. The challenge of weight loss isn't always pretty, and you've been a great husband through it all.

We especially would like to thank Judy Linden for her help in the development of this book. Without her stumbling upon us, this book would not have been. Judy knew what the book could be, and she encouraged us to believe that we did have it in us. We also thank her for giving us Bev West and Judy Capodanno, to help us work together and make the best book we could.

Thank you to Mark Lockett, M.D., for his valuable help in providing a surgeon's insight into weight-loss surgery.

We would also like to thank the moderators of 3fatchicks.com and their constant help with 3FC and the many dieters who come our way looking for support and answers. These women are a fount of information, and without them, 3FC would not be what it is. All of these women work hard to make sure that all of us looking for answers get on the healthiest path that we possibly can. Thank you, Sherry Abernathy, Sandi Blair, Karen Canzoneri, Jane M. Catt, Eileen Cordes, Lauren B. Dale, Marti Dyche, Laurie A. Garner, Melanie Gumerman, Karen Kossowsky, Meg Heinz, Carol Lemon, Ellen McCorkle, Jane F. Perrotta, Amy M. Phillippe, Michelle Powell, Christina Preece, Ilene Robertson, Ruth Sheridan, Lianne Slaughter, and Geri Thueme.

Last but not least, we'd like to thank the members of 3fatchicks.com, for all you do in making 3FC a home for thousands of chicks across the globe.

contents

introduction
meet the fat chicks

Hi, WE'RE THE 3 FAT CHICKS, Suzanne, Jennifer, and Amy, three sisters of the South who have eaten enough empty calories among us in our lifetimes to drive old Dixie down. But not anymore. Because we're on a diet—again!

The truth is, we've been on a diet for most of our lives. We've tried them all, from Atkins to Weight Watchers, from the Ice Cream diet to Cabbage Soup, and everything in between. We've busted sugar, cut carbs, flushed fat, counted calories, and gorged on grapefruit. Secretly we dreamed of a diet that consisted exclusively of pecan pie, which we know was a little nutty, but hey, we're southerners and we believe in the miraculous potential of molasses and nutmeats.

Needless to say, we were somewhat less than successful in those early battles of the bulge, but now something has changed and that has made all the difference. That something is 3fatchicks.com.

We started 3fatchicks.com as a way for the three of us to track our own weight-loss progress. It introduced a little bit of accountability into our secret wars with our waistlines and gave us an opportunity to support and encourage one another, even when we were all alone in our own homes, with a bag of chips singing sweetly to us from the kitchen, daring us to eat just one!

The idea was that we would log our progress for better or worse, keep a written journal of our ups and downs, and post our favorite recipes and tips to help each other over the difficult moments, to help us just say no to the all-you-can-eat buffets of our former fat lives.

Imagine our surprise then, when our picture wound up in *USA To-day* alongside the address to our Web site! Suddenly our secret support group wasn't such a secret anymore. We had been "outed" as fat chicks, coast to coast!

At first we were mortified. Well, in our picture we were standing in front of an all-you-can-eat buffet sign, which is not exactly a flattering backdrop for three women in muumuus and maternity shorts who weren't expecting anything but a third trip to the buffet table. But our embarrassment soon turned to enthusiasm as other fellow soldiers fighting the battle of the bulge began flooding our site. They offered their thoughts and feelings, successes and failures, hints and horror stories, all in the hopes of helping us win the war with our weight. And suddenly we began to feel a little bit better about, well, just about everything. We realized that we weren't alone. Our unexpected spirit squad cheered us on when we lost weight, and when we gained an inch or two, they cheered even louder! Suddenly we had more support than we ever dreamed of, and we began to lose weight and keep it off, with a little help from our on-line friends.

3 Fat Chicks on a Diet takes our Web site one step further. We have rounded up former and current fat chicks from across the nation—everyone from stay-at-home moms to biker chicks to sweet sixteens to high-powered executives—and asked them to share their ideas about the ups and downs of the total dieting experience, not only calorically but emotionally and psychologically.

The women represented in this real-women's guide to dieting are short, tall, young, old, single, married, separated, and divorced, but they all have one thing in common: they want to be thinner. We have organized their straight talk and ours into a no-holds-barred book about what it's really like to wage a war over our own impulses and lose weight.

In this book you'll find the information that other diet books and the celebrity gurus won't tell you. Here are helpful pointers about the little things that the big diet books forget to mention and honest assessments of the most popular diets on the planet from the women who have really tried to follow them. The questions and answers in this book are all based on our own 3fatchicks.com forum discussions as well as a survey that was conducted with thousands of our visitors and members.

Best of all, this isn't a book that requires that you go from the first page to the last page. You can weave in and out and flip around to the section you like, just as at an all-you-can-eat buffet, only you won't have to loosen your pants when you're through! Now that's something to cluck about! We hope you enjoy our book and the fun—yes, *fun*—of dieting together.

Love,
The 3 Fat Chicks, Suzanne, Jennifer, and Amy

3 fat chicks
on a diet

welcome to
the henhouse

WHEN YOU'RE CONTEMPLATING a climb up the slippery slope of weight loss toward your personal fitness peak, it's best not to spend too much time looking up at the steep trail ahead. When you look too far up the path in front of you, it's very easy to get winded just thinking about the climb, then turn around and go back to the lodge for a hot chocolate topped with a double scoop of "I'll start my diet tomorrow." But we did find it enormously helpful, when we started on our personal weight-loss journeys, to take in a quick view from the summit, through the eyes of somebody who has been there, to give ourselves the inspiration and the confidence to set out for the top.

The three of us have started more diets than Richard Petty has started races. We are sisters trying to drop over a hundred pounds apiece who don't have chefs, daily visits from our personal trainer, or elaborate home gyms. We understand what it's like to go it alone, without paid staff or even, in some cases, much support from our family and friends. And perhaps most important, we've learned that very few of us go on a diet and just lose weight. We also have to shed a lot of excess emotional baggage.

Most successful weight loss usually involves taking a long look at ourselves, making decisions to change the way we feel about ourselves and our eating habits, and discovering what success really means to us as individuals. This can be a very lonely experience at times, and for us, the help, support, and encouragement we got from each other and from our 3FC family made all the difference over the long haul. Hearing from women like us, who knew that learning how to just say no to a Big Mac can feel like nothing short of a religious conversion, made things easier. It really helped to know that we weren't alone, that there were women up on the trail ahead of us, who had found a way to climb beyond the world of pizza and popcorn and mac-and-cheese cravings and achieve their goal weight.

So for all of you chicks down there in the base camp getting ready for your final ascent, we'd like to share our three stories and the experiences of some very inspirational women, as well as the five most important steps we've identified that can prepare you for a successful climb. We hope our stories will fuel your motivation and your imagination, inspiring you to keep on going and never, never, never give up.

Jennifer 3FC

I've had weight issues almost all my life. I was probably a chubby fetus. My dieting experience started early. When I was eight years old, my doctor said I needed to lose weight, and he told my mother to water down my milk. Great idea! I went home and had a glass of watered-down milk with a Little Debbie cake!

Chubby girls aren't usually the most popular kids in school. I had only a few friends, but I made up for that with new friends, like Mr. Goodbar, Ronald McDonald, and Her Majesty the Dairy Queen. I was lonely, but that was okay, because it gave me plenty of time to snack.

Then hormones hit and I discovered boys, pimples, and PMS. My weight evened out. I sprouted boobs and a few curves. However, most of the other girls still had boyish figures, and I was fooled into thinking I was fat. As a gullible teenager, I tried every diet that was hot. I tried cabbage soup diets, grapefruit diets, fasting diets, negative calorie diets, and a tasty vinegar-water and kelp diet that I can still taste when I think about it.

When I moved out of my parents' house, I could no longer afford fancy luxury foods like fruits and vegetables. I lived on rice, noodles, bread, and whatever fatty meat I could find in the death row section of the meat department. I steadily gained up until pregnancy. Now I was knocked up, and so was my appetite, and I ballooned.

Finally, when my sisters and I started 3 Fat Chicks on a Diet, *I began to make some real changes in my lifestyle and my attitude toward food and health. I've spent years playing tag with my metabolism. Now I've caught up to myself, and most important, I've developed reasonable expectations. I don't want to be a skinny chick. I don't want to be a fat chick. I want to be a curvy chick. I just want to be me, and for the first time since I was eight years old, I finally feel like that's okay.*

Amy 3FC

There is something about me in a kitchen that just spells trouble. I could write the textbook for Cooking Disasters 101. I almost caught my house on fire while broiling a steak. I didn't realize there was something called a broiler pan. Who knew? Then I was evicted from an apartment after forgetting about a pan of boiling eggs that exploded all over the ceiling. Experiences like these led me to develop a close relationship with my local pizza delivery boy. He was always punctual, he required nothing of me besides a tip, cleanup was a breeze, ordering out saved me a load of time, and most important, nothing ever ignited. Unfortunately, my cooking alternative was also addictive and extremely fattening.

I did try to lose weight, and my choice of diets was as quick and easy as the dinners that got me there in the first place. I devised the "nothing but one Whopper a day" diet. I went on a laxative diet and a five-hundred-calorie a day diet. I mixed Slim-Fast with water instead of milk to save calories. My quick weight-loss schemes destroyed my metabolism quicker than one of those exploding eggs destroyed my ceiling. The more I dieted, the slower I lost weight. How's that for frustrating?

After I remarried, I found myself in the middle of a southern-fried Brady Bunch *episode. I was a newlywed and my husband delighted me daily with feasts big enough for a family of seven. Then suddenly that honeymoon was over, and that's when I developed a relationship with the Chi-*

nese buffet restaurant in town, and my weight blossomed faster than a magnolia grove in springtime. Finally, though, my quick fixes began to seriously impact my health.

I began to collect illnesses quicker than I did two-for-one pizza coupons, and I finally admitted that I'd lost control and I had to do something drastic. At nearly three hundred pounds I bit the bullet and had gastric bypass surgery. For the first time in more than twenty years, I am in control, I'm healthy, I'm confident. I've lost my delivery boys' phone numbers, and most miraculous of all, I've learned how to work a broiler pan!

Suzanne 3FC

My transition from a skinny kid to a fat chick was painless. I moved into my first apartment when I was eighteen years old, and for the first time I could eat anything I wanted to eat, whenever I felt like it. And I did! Breakfast was frosting on a spoon, lunch was chips and dip, and dinners always concluded with an Oreo-thon that went on late into the night. Sure, I got pudgy, but I was enjoying every white, creamy middle and chocolate cookie outside along the way.

As the years went on, my menus were dictated less by impulse than budget. When things were good, I experimented with recipes from Gourmet magazine. When things were tough, I lived on mac and cheese. Rich or poor, I was always loaded with calories, which obviously resulted in weight gain. When I became a single parent, with a stressful job, my life was made easier by the help of a personal chef who always wore red and yellow and never forgot to ask if I wanted to super-size it. By the time I reached my early thirties, I was a full-fledged fat chick, but for some reason I did not consider dieting. I just ignored the situation. When the day finally came that I felt the urge to double-check the load capacity of an elevator before stepping in with my sisters, I realized that I needed to do something drastic—like go on a diet. Since then, I have fired my personal chef, learned to cook healthy and delicious meals, and taken back control of my health—all because I finally stopped ignoring my problems.

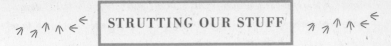

STRUTTING OUR STUFF

The Chicks Sound Off on Their Personal Last Straws

We asked some of our chicks about their memories of the last straw that finally convinced them to change their lives forever. As you read through these snapshots, ask yourself what the first day of the rest of your life might be like. Maybe it's today!

I got really out of breath trying to tie my tennis shoes and realized that I wasn't even forty years old and if I can't breathe to tie my shoes now, what's it going to be like ten years from now? — CHAR

My mom came out for an extended visit from California a few years ago. It started off with me pretending, while my mom was visiting, that I don't usually eat like a pig. It ended with me realizing that I had dropped a few pounds while she was here and that the choice was mine whether to continue or not. It was a turning point, and at the time I didn't fully appreciate the magnitude of my power of choice. Now I can't help but wonder: what if I had chosen a different path? That thought alone is enough to make me put my fork down when I should, or go exercise when I really don't feel like it, and maintain my accomplishment. — BEVERLY

I had to go to a funeral. I had two pairs of black pants, a size 8 and a size 12. I didn't even consider the 8s. The 12s were the kind that button inside the pockets. I had already moved the buttons once, but that day they didn't even reach the holes anymore. I had to loop an elastic band through the buttonhole and around the last button and keep my coat on through the whole funeral. That day at the funeral buffet, I had a black

• *Continued on next page* •

decaf. By the end of the month I was walking every day. The rest is history. —SUSAN

On the way back from a three-week trip to England, I couldn't zip my size 18 jeans for the return flight, and I felt dreadful for the entire time. Ten hours flying in coach in jeans two sizes too small changed my life forever. —MEL

The Five Essential Steps to Long-Term Weight Loss

1. Find a Support System

No chick is an island. You can't lose weight without a shoulder to lean on, so put a support system in place before taking the big leap. If you're not getting support from your family, find a new family. Seriously, there are options even if your family is less than enthusiastic about the bunless burgers that have begun to appear on the dinner table. Consider joining Weight Watchers, or look for a local support group at a hospital or church. Find walking buddies in the neighborhood, arrange your budget to accommodate gym fees, join an on-line support group, or visit 3fatchicks.com!

Howie and Kimberley are partners in diet and marriage. Between them, they've lost more than 250 pounds. Kimberley has lost 50 pounds, and Howie has lost 202 pounds, and they each have about 50 pounds to go. They have found that embarking on this journey together has helped them get through the tough times. The way they applaud and encourage each other is truly an inspiration to us all, and the perfect example of the kind of solid support system you'll want to try to develop. Not all of us are lucky enough to have a partner to succeed with, but having anybody in life who's there to pick you up when you stumble is a tremendous help. Here's what Kimberley and Howie had to say about the importance of their mutual support system.

Kimberley

Howie and I have dieted together off and on over the course of our marriage. The fact that he's my best friend helps a lot, and we can be either our own worst enemies or our own best coaches when it comes to weight loss. Having a partner, be it a spouse, friend, or another family member, really helps. Having 3FC and friends here helps us to stay accountable too. I have realized through this process that it isn't just my weight that's important, but my health. I love life, I love my husband, and I want to be healthy.

Howie

I have now lost over two hundred pounds from my heaviest. What a feeling! It is so much easier doing this with my best friend. She gives me strength to go on when I'm feeling weak. I am so proud of her for the weight she has lost and I know she will follow through with this to the end. I can't wait to see what we feel like when we lose "another person."

I really admire Kimberley for sticking to this even though the weight has been coming off really slowly for her. She is doing so well and is such a help to me. It makes it a lot easier when you have someone to make this trip with.

2. Load Up on Self-Esteem

A lack of self-esteem can wreck any chance you have at weight loss. Hating yourself really doesn't help the pounds come off. And remember, confidence doesn't have any calories. Before undertaking a serious weight-loss program, you need to heal yourself emotionally. Imagine if you were responsible for giving first aid to two people— one you hated and one you loved. Who would get the better care? Give that same care to yourself.

This means accepting yourself as you are, not as you wish you were. You're overweight: get over it. Everybody knows you're overweight, so there's no sense in trying to hide it. Accept who you are, and enjoy the fact that this will help you in your weight loss. Jessica, also known on our forum as Goddess Jessica, gives us some golden ways to learn how to love yourself.

Jessica

I had such a skewed idea of my body, so I took some examples from anorexic therapy books. See, anorexics think they are way bigger than they are. (Remind you of anybody?) Therapy includes a ton of very helpful exercises. Here are some things I do:

- *Get in front of the camera. A lot! Post pictures of yourself around areas of low self-esteem, such as the scale, the closet. I had this idea that I was so big that Geraldo was going to have to pry my walls off to get me out of the house. That is such a crock.*

- *Find some positive things to look at in the mirror. I had a huge problem getting out of the shower and feeling bad about myself. Now I wiggle and jiggle in front of the mirror, practicing my bedroom eyes and such. But also look at those areas you hate to look at. Quit imagining how bad they are and look. Yep, I'm fat, but I've got the nicest hourglass figure anyone could ask for.*

- *Finally, get out and do something you shouldn't do for a "woman of your size." I took belly dancing classes. Heck, I have a belly, shouldn't I use it? Gain some confidence for doing something you didn't think you'd enjoy doing. Then do it again!*

I'm lucky. I had a bad mental image of myself but lots of confidence. Now I'm reconciling the two.

3. Find a Less-Fattening Form of Comfort

We all have different reasons for needing an emotional rescue, but when we're on a diet, our answers can't be cream-filled or dipped in glaze anymore. Jane, one of the 3FC moderators, decided to get serious about her weight loss in January 2004. She is just fifteen pounds away from her goal weight and has maintained her diet because she learned how to reward herself without indulging in the comfort of empty calories. Here's what Jane had to say about combating her head hunger.

Jane

In order to finally lose the weight and keep it off, I had to find out what I personally got as a reward from staying overweight. For me, it was the comfort of eating. I used food to calm my nerves, soothe my bruised feelings, and also to celebrate. The way these foods made me feel was my payoff, so I had to find a different way to get the same satisfaction. My answer was limiting my portions, or finding a different kind of reward system, like an hour of junk TV instead of junk food, or going for long walks, or taking some time to tend to my garden when I needed a little comfort. The next thing I did was to enlist the support of my family. Also I got all the junk food out of my house. Yes, I can, and do, have treats, but a steady supply of them is just too tempting.

I have noticed in the past that when I lose for a specific event, such as a wedding, a reunion, or a vacation, I always gain the weight right back after the event is over. So this time I am losing for the rest of my life. Until the day I die, I will be doing Weight Watchers, because I want to!

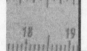

filling the void

Here are some tips from our chicks on how they overcame emotional eating:

Keep a journal and write down every bite that passes through your lips, and why you ate it. Even if you're pissed at the world, you're not likely to let that list get filled with unhealthy foods. —MARIA, VERMONT

I go to bed each night before I get too tired. I find that when I get sleepy, that is when I nibble, trying to stay alert to read or watch TV.

● Continued on next page ●

I'm less likely to eat bags of popcorn and frozen pizza at 7 A.M.!
—JULIA, TEXAS

I stay busy when my husband is away. I tend to nibble on bad things that I'd never dream of eating in front of him. I make sure when he is going to be away that I plan a project to keep my hands busy or go out with friends. —DONNA, VIRGINIA

4. Discover Something You Love and Stick with It

When you're feeling deprived on a diet, try thinking about the things that you are adding to your life, rather than the things that you are subtracting, like pecan pie and pizza. Change can be hard to get used to. By focusing on the positive, you'll find yourself feeling better about saying no to those empty calories, and success will come a lot easier. Rubia, one of our forum members, has taught us that successful weight loss is not about giving things up but about finding new and healthier ways to excite your passion for living.

Rubia
I'm five seven and since my teens I've always weighed around 160 pounds. When I went away to college I gained 35 pounds in nine months. I was a mess. My clothes didn't fit; I was depressed and looked like a whole different person. One day I watched a step aerobics class and decided to give it a shot. I absolutely loved it! I've been addicted to step ever since. I lost that 35-pound weight gain, then I went on vacation and somehow lost 10 more pounds! I realized I didn't always have to be 160 pounds. I was looking better, clothes were fitting me better, and I felt great! When people ask me for advice, I always say find something you love to do, and then do it as often as you can. There is something out there for all of us.

5. Try Gradual Change Instead of Going Cold Turkey

Weight loss isn't easy, but it can seem harder than it really is. We all know someone who has quit smoking cold turkey, but dieting is rarely that simple. If you are used to a certain kind of food, or lack of activity, it can seem daunting to change your habits and dive into a new diet and fitness program.

Change can be hard to get used to, so it's sometimes better to start off with small changes, rather than beating yourself up because you can't do it all at once. Focus on one meal a day and make that meal healthier. Wear a pedometer and try to add a few hundred more steps each day. By focusing on the small changes, you'll find yourself feeling better about yourself, and the rest will come a lot easier!

Jennifer, one of our forum members, has taught us that successful weight loss doesn't have to be instant, or an all-or-nothing venture. She decided it would be easier to concentrate on one small change at a time. Jennifer made little changes that would improve her health, such as adding a new vegetable to her diet or replacing white rice with brown. Jennifer even took her weight-loss goals slowly, making small goals of ten pounds at a time. These gradual changes helped make losing weight, and getting healthier, virtually painless. She soon realized there was nothing to stop her from reaching her goals.

Jennifer

I made "rules for myself" for weight loss. One of the top rules is that there will be no radical, unsustainable changes. When I first decided I wanted to change my eating habits to be stronger and healthier, I knew I needed something I could stick with forever. I couldn't radically change how I eat: there's no way to maintain that long term. With my boyfriend's support, we started changing foods one at a time to get used to our new, healthier eating habits. I am also making small changes toward exercise, which I do not like! I've taken the first baby steps by joining a gym.

Since I originally started, I got a tattoo to help me stay focused and committed. The tattoo is a Chinese proverb that means, "Dripping water can eat through stone," to help me remember it's every tiny step that leads to success. It is very meaningful to me: it represents all the hard work I've done this year. I have never given up, not for one second. I kept making changes, both big and little, to be the healthiest person I can be.

how not to diet

We totally understand the lure of easy weight loss. What chick isn't blinded by the sentence "Lose ten pounds in three days"? Amazing weight-loss claims are a sure sign that a diet isn't healthy or that it doesn't promote fat loss. If you really want to know if a product works, ask your doctor—not the savvy marketers who wrote the testimonials and product claims. Remember, if diet pills, gadgets, and miracle diets worked like they claimed, our doctors and insurance companies would be pushing them on us. We'd hear about them on CNN, not infomercials and e-mail spam. And America wouldn't be the most obese country on the planet.

- **Over-the-counter diet pills.** If you need a diet pill, get it from your doctor, not from a truck stop or flea market stall. Some contain properties that could be harmful to your body— particularly your heart. The fine print always tells you to go on a reduced-calorie diet and exercise program. That's how you lose the weight.
- **Weight-loss jewelry, clothing, and shoes.** We don't care how many women in the ads claim to have kept slim with these products. Believe us, a pinky ring will not make your butt smaller.
- **Diet patches.** These usually contain various herbs that won't help you lose weight and may not even be absorbed through your skin anyway. The only way a diet patch can help you lose weight is if you use it to tape your mouth shut.
- **Extreme diet schemes.** Cabbage soup, grapefruit, water, and juice diets might sound good in theory, but after three days of eating nothing but citrus fruit, it starts to get a little difficult to unpucker, and cabbage, well, let's just say cabbage can

be a little windy when eaten in mass quantities. Also, unbalanced meals like these do nothing for you nutritionally. Limiting your foods to only one type can be harmful, not to mention boring, and so can extremely low-calorie diets. Our bodies need protein, carbohydrates, and fat to thrive. The only thing you really wind up losing on these crash diets is your sense of humor.

- **"Detox" plans.** That's just a fancy version of Ex-Lax and a jug of water. There is no scientific evidence that "detoxing" will help you lose weight, but it has been proven in extreme cases to cause coma or even death. Besides, if you were truly toxic, you'd need a trip to the ER, not the health food store. Make water and fiber a part of your healthy diet to keep your system clean. If you are concerned, please ask your doctor for advice.
- **Diets that claim you'll lose weight effortlessly.** That's just not how it works. If it did, we'd all be running around in size 2 bikinis. Weight loss takes a change in lifestyle, through diet and exercise.

Picking the diet that works for you is one of the most important first steps in successful weight loss, but how do you pick from the wide array of plans available today? Before you put all your eggs into one diet basket, take some time to listen to what our chicks have to say about the most popular programs around. In the pages to come, you'll hear from real chicks who have been eating on the beach, dining with Dr. Atkins, or counting their points on Weight Watchers. Their candid thoughts about what worked for them and what didn't, along with answers to their most frequently asked questions, troubleshooting suggestions, helpful hints, and personal stories about the agony and the ecstasy of weight loss, will help you figure out which program is right for you. The questions addressed in these chapters are based on our own forum discussions as well as a survey that was conducted with thousands of our visitors and members. The answers are designed to give you the real-world information, support, and insight that you will need to ride the crest of those crave waves all the way to the shores of better health. Make the diet you choose this time your last.

Words to Live By

I have gained and lost the same ten pounds so many times over and over again, my cellulite must have déjà vu. —JANE WAGNER

To eat is a necessity, but to eat intelligently is an art.
—LA ROCHEFOUCAULD

fat chicks on the beach
the south beach diet

T HE SOUTH BEACH DIET is one of the most misunderstood diets in the coop because everybody thinks it's a variation on the low-carb philosophy of the Atkins diet. Well, we fat chicks on the beach are here to tell you that the South Beach diet is not *at all* like the Atkins plan. This diet limits the types of carbs, not the amount, and also limits the types of fats you eat, which makes for a very different dieting experience.

Unlike Atkins, the South Beach diet does allow a few glorious carbs. But don't get too excited. South Beach–friendly carbs aren't exactly the carbs we dieting-down-in-Dixie chicks know and love. There will be no French fries, or fritters, no pound cake or pralines, and definitely no Moon Pies.

Basically, on the South Beach plan, you're not going to eat anything white or greasy (including anything named Bubba). No white potatoes, white bread, white rice, sugar (white *or* brown), or white flour. But here's the kicker. Unlike the Atkins plan, the South Beach diet limits your fat in addition to your carbohydrates. This means no full-fat dairy, no bacon or standard oils with a lot of saturated fats either. Ready to turn to the next chapter?

Well, hang on a minute, there is some good news . . .

You *are* allowed to eat a whole lot of earth tones on the beach. You can eat some bread and even rice, as long as they're brown and whole-grain. And you can eat some potatoes too, so long as they're sweet potatoes (which make delicious french fries, by the way, simmered in a little monounsaturated fat). You can also eat olive oil, nuts, avocados, lean meats, veggies, and most fruits. Is your mouth watering yet? Ours isn't either, but remember, this is a diet that was originally devised to maintain heart health, so it's very good for more than maintaining your waistline: it improves your overall health and can even increase your longevity. And because it is a more balanced diet than Atkins, it's an easier and healthier plan to maintain long-term. Are those sweet potatoes starting to sound a little better now? Well, read on.

Dr. Arthur Agatston, a cardiologist, who could be called the accidental millionaire, developed the South Beach diet (SBD) to help improve his patients' cardiac health. Coincidentally, the diet was also very effective for weight loss. His patients lost weight, felt great, and shared their secret with friends. This plan was probably passed around Southern Florida on folded-up photocopies, just like the "Mayo" diet from the eighties, which wasn't really from the Mayo Clinic at all. But who cares about pedigree if it works?

On the South Beach diet you can eat three meals plus snacks each day, and you don't have to count calories, which is good, because who can do math when they're woozy with carb and fat depletion? The South Beach diet does have one very important rule: *stop eating when you aren't hungry anymore.* While moderation might seem like an obvious boundary, for most of us fat chicks on the beach, overeating is what made us fat in the first place, so learning when to say no to seconds and thirds is a little tricky. Once you master this simple rule of thumb, though, the South Beach diet is very effective long-term, and remarkably easy to follow.

The South Beach diet is divided into three phases. Phase 1, which lasts for two weeks, restricts most carbs and most fat. As we carb- and fat-aholics can attest, when you first hit the South Beach surf, it can feel like a real diet tidal wave, and the level of restriction has knocked more than a few of us off our boards. One bad case of the Krispy Kreme blues, and you can find yourself caught in the undertow and wind up miles from the beach before you even realize it. And then sometimes you have to start all over again. After an experience like this, a lot of chicks decide to go in search of friendlier diet waters. In fact, in a recent poll we conducted on 3fatchicks.com, 75 percent of us who wound up quitting the diet quit during Phase 1. So hold on through this early phase as long as you can, and try your best not to get frustrated. And more important, be realistic. The Fat Fairy didn't zap the pounds on overnight, so shedding them might take some time. If you stick with the program during Phase 1 boot camp though, you can lose up to thirteen pounds in just two weeks! Now that's what we call a hang ten!

If you make it through these two weeks, you will be rewarded with Phase 2, when the diet becomes much easier. Phase 2 allows additional complex carbohydrates and monounsaturated fats. So you *can* have your cake and eat it too, but only if that cake is made with whole-wheat flour and olive oil.

Phase 3 of the South Beach diet is designed for long-term maintenance. During this phase, you add more foods so that you stop losing weight but don't gain any pounds back either. Basically, Phase 3 is like Phase 2, only with larger portions. Phase 3 of the South Beach diet is no longer a weight-loss diet but a new way of eating that you will continue with for as long as you wish to remain at your goal weight—which is probably forever!

As with any weight-loss plan, there are issues with the South Beach diet that make it, well, a diet. Some of the issues cause dieters to give up too easily or, like some of us do, stick with it but bitch all the way. So it's not surprising that our community of South Beach beauties had very strong emotional responses to this diet. Those of us who thrive on a sense of control would reassure ourselves, at the end of a hectic and otherwise helpless day, that if nothing else, we managed to stay on program. Some of us recognized that we would sooner stick needles in our eyes than say good-bye to spuds and abandoned the beach for a diet that understood that sometimes french fries are two dozen of the best reasons to get out of bed in the morning.

In our responses we grappled with being so close, yet so far away from that real piece of cake. We struggled with food charts and meal planning, carb cravings, headaches, and feelings of inadequacy when we didn't lose as much weight as quickly as we had hoped. We really would have preferred the pounds to come off as enjoyably and deliciously as we packed them on!

So for all of you chicks who have just hit the beach, or for those who are thinking about rolling up your blanket and calling it a day, below is the collective wisdom of our fat chicks on the beach, who have made it through Phase 1, broken through the boredom of Phase 2, and reached their weight-loss goals.

meet the fat chicks on the beach

Laurie from New York

I once weighed 326 pounds (or more!). My ankles were swollen, I was out of breath, and I structured my life at home around avoiding the stairs because climbing them was too painful. I had terrible pain in my back, hips, shoulders, and ribs, and it took about five minutes of excruciating pain for my back to straighten out when I lay down at night. I had increasingly bad cholesterol, blood pressure, and heart rate, and I had a terrible self-image. On top of it all, my husband and I wanted to get pregnant, and I knew there was no way I was ever going to be able to healthily become pregnant at that weight. I picked up a copy of The South Beach Diet *at Wal-Mart one night after my doctor recommended it. I was thinking I would look it over, just to see, but my husband was very excited that I had bought it, so I figured I might as well try it. Now I'm healthier than I've been in more than a decade. I work out and all of the problems mentioned above are either much improved or completely gone.*

Jane from Arizona
I had been low-carbing on and off for a few years but I found that I gained immediately after even the tiniest "cheats" and I never figured out a way around them. I decided South Beach might work better for me, and it did! I'm so thrilled! I love it!

Amy from Michigan
When I first started the South Beach diet, I did everything exactly like it's written in the book. And you definitely need the book to do this diet successfully. I never ate any more or less for the first two weeks and I dropped 16.5 pounds and I was thrilled. This diet taught me that not only what you eat matters but also how much of what you eat. Portion control has made this a very successful plan for me.

Q: *I'm a week into Phase 1 of the South Beach diet, I'm tired all the time, I don't feel any skinnier, and my cravings are so intense that I'd trade my first-born for a cheeseburger deluxe. Help!*

3FC: The good news is that you aren't the first South Beach beauty who wanted a warm, soft bun so much she'd seduce Ronald himself to get it. We have all seen our families freeze like deer in the headlights when we walk through the door at suppertime with that look in our eye. We've all found ourselves growling at our pooch when he gets near his dog biscuits. And we've all looked up and actually seen the word *surrender* forming in the clouds above our aching heads. But don't worry, Dorothy, you're not in Oz, you're in Phase 1, and unfortunately the only answer is, *Do not give up.*

What you're going through is called carb detox, and we know it's not pretty. Carb detox is difficult, but the upshot of going through it is that once you cleanse your system, you won't feel those cravings anymore. You'll be free from carb addiction and actually crave healthier foods, the same way that you're craving that Big Mac right now.

Think of Phase 1 as hazing session at a frat party, minus the part where you have to wear underwear on your head. It might be difficult at the moment, but enduring this brief humiliation pays you back with a lifetime of membership privileges. Once your blood sugar stabilizes, your cravings will go away. For most people, the side effects only last a week or two. Would Scarlett have given up on Tara in two weeks? We don't think so. So when the going gets tough, remember: Phase 1, like everything in life except death, taxes, and dryer lint, shall pass.

In the meantime, if it gets too bad, just lock yourself in a room and have your family slide omelets and turkey rollups under the door while you watch *Super Size Me* over and over from the safety of your bedroom. And when you feel like you just can't hold out another moment, try our bacon cheeseburger salad on page 38 or a few of the detox remedies our fellow beach beauties have found to help you get through those long, hard, carbless nights when you're afraid you're going to rush out and mug the pizza delivery boy.

detox remedies for recovering carbo-holics in crisis

- One sure way to kill a carb craving is sugar-free Jell-O. We're not talking about the little sundae dish of Jell-O cubes with a dainty dollop of fat-free whipped cream. We want you to make a few boxes of the stuff, just litter the fridge with big bowls of multihued Jell-O. Then, when you can't go a moment longer without a carb or sugar fix, raid the fridge. And we mean *really* dig in, like a liposuction machine in reverse. Jell-O is sweet and it's filling, and if you eat it without moaning, you'll probably hear the choir of angels singing in the background.

- Take a nap. You're still allowed to eat carbs in your dreams.
- Drink a lot of water. You need to flush your system, and water will give you the illusion of being full.
- Play Scrabble. Spell words like *coronary, plaque, muumuu,* or *obese.*
- Get the most bang for your buck with sugar-free Fudgsicles, hot cocoa, and hazelnut syrup for your coffee. These are long-lasting treats; by the time you have finished them, the cravings will be gone.
- We suggest snacks, snacks, and more snacks! You need a few extra munchies when you are kicking the cravings in the beginning. Try almonds, low-fat cheese sticks, sugar-free Jell-O, or fresh veggies and lean lunchmeats. Salad veggies and a good dressing low in saturated fat are very important! And since you are living with people you care for, until those early cravings pass, we'd suggest sedatives and a padded room!
- Here's a good dip for your turkey rollups: Find a jar of tapenade. It's a thick spread made of olives, olive oil, and spices. Mix a heaping tablespoon of tapenade with one ounce of light cream cheese that's been softened a bit. This is a *wonderful* dip or spread for your turkey rollups!

Q: Breakfast is boring me to death. Every morning is eggs, eggs, eggs, and more eggs. I have been doing the first phase of SBD and am very happy with the program. But I have eaten so many eggs in one week that I feel like I really will turn into a chicken. I am in grad school and have class every morning at 8 A.M. and I have a forty-five-minute commute, so cooking a big breakfast every morning just isn't cutting it anymore. Help!

3FC: Breakfast is a killer. And when you're cutting carbs, you can find yourself eating so many eggs that you'll make them scrambled just for the pure pleasure of beating them with a blunt object. Eggs get old *real* fast. Fortunately, eggs are very versatile and forgiving, and with the right combination of ingredients, you can totally fool your rebellious taste buds into believing that they are sensing something fabulous! So before you move on to explore a beach without eggs, try a few of our recipes for eggs with a twist on pages 35–36.

Of course, you don't even have to eat traditional breakfast foods. Sticking to traditional foods shows a worker-bee attitude. You can be a rebel and try something totally different! Make up a batch of chicken salad, tuna salad, shrimp salad, or (if you really have a hard time breaking tradition) egg salad made with low-fat mayonnaise. Fill a romaine lettuce leaf or two, and you have a quick and tasty breakfast.

If you'd like something warm and rich for breakfast, try reheating a vegetable casserole, or even the crab cake recipe from the official South Beach cookbook. It doesn't have to be limited to dinner. Try a crab cake for breakfast, and start your day in the lap of luxury! You can also have a spicy chicken breast or even a bowl of warm black bean soup with salsa and fat-free sour cream on top. We also like veggie burgers for breakfast, with a smear of mustard and tomato on top. Diets are a lot like life. The key to happiness is to think outside the box. Think of what you *can* have and don't focus on what you can *not* have. With that perspective, the possibilities are endless!

STRUTTING OUR STUFF

I often eat last night's leftovers if they appeal to me, or sometimes I'll have cottage cheese, low-fat cheese, or lunchmeat rollups and V-8 juice. Once you are on Phase 2, you can have things like a fat-free yogurt blended with berries, Splenda, and vanilla. —MARTHA IN OHIO

Sometimes I just grab a couple of slices of low-fat cheese and a handful of nuts when I can't face cooking. Mostly I have eggs and cheese or low-fat sausages with mushrooms or tomatoes, or I'll make quiche cups ahead of time, for a quick and easy breakfast. —FRANK IN WASHINGTON

If I'm running late, I usually have a V-8 and cheese sticks, or what I call an Egg McNuthin. (Buy an Egg McMuffin, and throw out the muffin!)—BONNIE IN IDAHO

Q: Is it healthy to cut out a food group in Phase 1? My mother always told me I should eat my fruit and bread!

3FC: Now, we know that Mother always knows best, and most of our mothers taught us from an early age to eat a well-balanced diet that included all four major food groups. If we didn't, they told us, our eating habits would lead to a lot of unladylike symptoms, such as bad breath, poor complexion, and slow bowels. Of course, in our family, one of those food groups was pecan pie, so we've learned to take Mom's menu suggestions with a grain of salt. Let's not forget that many of our moms also taught us that a balanced lunch included a PB&J on fluffy white Wonder bread, an apple, and a glass of whole milk. So it's no wonder, then, that Phase 1 of the South Beach diet, which eliminates fruit and bread and severely limits dairy, can cause us to feel fundamentally uneasy, as if we're breaking the Ten Commandments of food. This has caused a lot of chicks to flee before finishing Phase 1. Apparently they never heard of Phase 2.

You need to remember that the unbalanced diet of Phase 1 only lasts two weeks. You're eating not to build strong bodies twelve ways but to cleanse your system from carbs and sugars. Once you get into Phase 2, you'll be able to gradually add fruits and whole grains back into your diet, along with more dairy products. The only thing you'll eliminate will be high-glycemic carbs and trans fats. Until you get to the end of Phase 1, you can improve your vitamin consumption with alternative foods that are on the Phase 1 program. Add vitamin C with broccoli, cauliflower, or bell peppers. You can increase your fiber with carbs such as black beans and fibrous vegetables from the Phase 1 list. Hang in there until Phase 1 has passed. Then you can safely invite your mother over for a nice sandwich on whole-wheat bread, washed down with a glass of nonfat milk, and we're sure she'll approve!

alternachick tips: vegetarians on the beach

The menu on the average reduced-carb diet is a vegetarian's nightmare. It's much easier on South Beach. Vegetarians follow the same plan as everyone else on South Beach, except in the choice of protein, and some of which may be limited due to fat or carb content.

Read the labels! You can have soy-based meat substitutes, but they can have no more than six grams of fat per two- or three-ounce serving. Others may contain rice or other ingredients not allowed during Phase 1.

My husband loves Mexican food, but my choices are obviously limited now. When we eat out, I choose the vegetable fajitas, without the tortilla. The filling is full of flavor, and they don't mind filling up my plate. Just double-check that the fajitas are not fried in lard! —JILL

I couldn't wait to reach Phase 2 so I could eat oatmeal with walnuts sprinkled on top. It has a bit of protein, some good omega-3 fats, and a powerhouse of heart-disease-fighting oats. —RUBY

I hate to cook and loved the convenience of tofu marinated in teriyaki or other sauces. Most contain sugar, so I had to learn how to season my own tofu, without sugary sauces, and avoid the premarinated kinds. —JEN

Q: I'm at the end of Phase 1, and I didn't lose eight to thirteen pounds like the book said I would! I feel like such a failure and I'm ready to give up!

3FC: Okay, so Phase 1 didn't move the earth and the sky for you. The book jacket said you could lose up to thirteen pounds, but you weren't even close. Welcome to Marketing 101. We read the same book jacket as you did, and it gave us the same funny feeling in our stomachs that we had when Publishers Clearing House told us we might *already* be millionaires! While there are certainly a couple of fortunate folks out there who did open their front door to find Ed McMahon standing there with a big fat check in his hand, most of us eventually have to face the fact that we are going to have to earn our luck the hard way. While it is true that dieters *might* lose eight to thirteen pounds in Phase 1, many of our South Beach beauties lost much less. But just because you weren't a big loser in Phase 1 doesn't make you a loser. Dieters who haven't been on a diet recently or haven't been watching their carb intake or those who are very overweight are the ones who drop the most weight in Phase 1.

In other words, the fatter you are, the more weight you lose up front. So if you didn't lose very much weight in Phase 1, it could just mean that you didn't have that much to lose! Keep in mind too that this early weight loss is mostly due to water lost because of your body's sudden drop in excess carbs. If you were already watching carbs, or if you had less excess water to spare, then you won't have as much water weight to shed. After all, there is only so much weight a fat chick can whiz away.

And of course, it's important to level with yourself. Are you sure that you ate everything on the plan to the letter? Are you sure there weren't any Mallomars moments that you've conveniently forgotten about? Did you really exercise, or was your activity confined to remote control curls and the occasional jog to the refrigerator? Did you drink enough fluids? Were you poaching chicken or makin' bacon?

Other common Phase 1 beach beauty blunders include eating too many nuts, eating cheese that was not low-fat, having too much dairy, or indulging in too many two-for-one cocktails at happy hour. Some of our beach beauties have discovered that journaling daily food intake makes a big difference. Try writing down every bite that you eat. You might be able to pinpoint where things went wrong, and correct those problems before they slow you down where it really counts—in Phase 2, and over the long haul.

deep thoughts from our heavy hens

The main thing I have learned through my weight-loss journey is that there are two major components: consistent exercise and the support of people who are in the same boat as you. —JENNIFER MOORE

The scariest thing about embarking on this journey is that I have no idea where it will end. In my entire life I have never been thin or even at a healthy weight. I was overweight as a child and have been that way all through my teenage years. Even when I lost weight in the past, I still remained in the "obese" category. So I don't even know how it's going to feel! I'm scared that once I start feeling good, I'll stop because I won't know how much better I could still feel. —RISHE

For the first time in my personal history, I'm hoping that my weight loss will be a by-product of changing my relationship with food, rather than

of dieting to lose the weight. I've had a dysfunctional relationship with food for most of my life. Breaking up with that has been liberating, and even if no weight loss occurs, I've already made the biggest change to help myself live a longer, healthier life. —AMY STEVENS

Q: Phase 1 just isn't working for me when it comes to lunch, because I am a sandwich freak. If I don't get my sandwich, somebody's gonna get hurt. Should I trash this diet?

3FC: Many dieters would chew off their left arm for a mere crumb of bread by the end of Phase 1. On the other side of the coin are those dieters who have the mutant ability to *not* crave carbs and who aren't quite ready to give up the rapid weight-loss regimen of Phase 1. For both ends of the carb cravings spectrum, we recommend that beach chicks consider what we call Phase 1.5. Phase 1.5 is completely unofficial. Phase 1.5 is basically Phase 1, with only one or two servings of Phase 2 carbs per day. It isn't full force, so you get the best of both worlds.

Q: I'm really reluctant to graduate from Phase 1! I am having a very hard time with that issue. I feel very good, my body is really trimming down (my husband is thrilled, as am I), and I am still enjoying the diet on Phase 1. I never really was a fruit eater, and I don't miss it. I suppose it might be nice to have an apple, but I don't really care. Also, I don't get all excited about whole grains. To me, what I can add in Phase 2 just sounds kind of boring, and I don't want to stall my weight loss. I know this sounds crazy, but can I just stay in Phase 1?

3FC: Dieting may not always be fun, but actually losing weight really is like one long, glorious day at the beach, and potentially one of the greatest experiences in your life. Knowing that you can make hard decisions and carry them out because it's the right thing to do for yourself is one of the best self-esteem builders around, but the only thing better than taking the weight off is keeping it off long-term. Phase 1 usually results in quick weight loss, and we lose more per week during this period than in Phase 2. So why would we want to give that up?

Well, because Phase 1 simply wasn't intended to be the whole diet, and it isn't nutritionally sound for long-term use. Phase 1 was intended to flush out water and get you past your carb cravings. If you are still having cravings, stay on it for another week or two, but no more. The name of the game here is better health. Besides, Phase 1 is primarily water loss, and there is only so much water you can shed! Staying on Phase 1 will not help you lose weight quicker, it will only burn you out.

Phase 2 is designed for healthy weight loss. You wouldn't want to continue to lose weight at the rate of Phase 1 anyway. That would be too hard on your body. Slowing down on the weight loss will give your skin a chance to catch up with your body and will keep your metabolism in balance. You wouldn't want to fool your body into thinking you were starving. If you eat too few calories, your body begins to believe it's going to be deprived long-term, and it begins to act like a squirrel gathering nuts for the winter. It will store your fat and save it for later. Unfortunately, later never comes, and we can wind up with a very full basement! So keeping your body nourished is as important on this diet as restricting your intake. If you do start to gain weight again on Phase 2, just cut back a little and you'll be fine. Be aware that a small gain may just be water, as your body replenishes part of what it lost in Phase 1.

To Market, to Market

Our Favorite Phase 2–Friendly Items

Let's face it, supermarkets can seem like a Shangri-La of forbidden fruits when you are starting out on a diet. And passing up

the potato chip pleasure dome for the produce aisle can be a
real exercise in self-control. So here's an easy rule of thumb: Do
not walk where even South Beach angels fear to tread. Most
South Beach–friendly food will come from the outer sections of
the grocery store. "Good carb" produce, lean meats and seafood, low-fat yogurts, cheeses, eggs, and quality deli meats are
usually arranged on the margins of the supermarket, which will
keep you out of the midsection, where they keep the Lay's and
the Chips Ahoy. Only dip into the tempting middle for grains,
condiments, and miscellaneous frozen foods. And while preparing food from scratch is the best way to ensure you don't have
hidden fats and carbs, we all know that there are times when we
just can't or don't want to cook. For times like these, here is a list
of our Chick Picks for the best South Beach–friendly prepared
foods easily found in your local grocery store.

- Uncle Sam's Cereal
  www.usmillsinc.com
- Smucker's Reduced Fat Natural Peanut Butter
  www.smuckers.com
- Pepperidge Farm 100% Whole Wheat Bread
  www.pepperidgefarm.com
- Bob's Red Mill Steel Cut Oats and Stone Ground Flour
  www.bobsredmill.com
- DaVinci Sugar Free Syrups
  www.davincigourmet.com
- Blue Bunny Health Smart Bars
  www.bluebunny.com
- Progresso Lentil Soup
  www.progressosoup.com
- Diet Rite with Splenda
  www.dietritecola.com
- Mission Whole Wheat Tortillas
  www.missionfoods.com

Q: Okay, I admit it. I'm a week into Phase 2, and I don't know what came over me, but last night I snuck into my kitchen when everyone was asleep and devoured three Boston cream doughnuts in the blink of an eye. I woke up with chocolate in my hair and Krispy Kreme remorse in my heart. Can I just forget about the whole thing and move on with Phase 2, or do I have to start over again from the very beginning and go back to Phase 1?

3FC: You can cheat on your husband, you can cheat on a test, and you can cheat on a diet. If you cheat on your diet, though, you have only to answer to yourself. The truth is you're going to feel inclined to cheat when you hear the word no. You've been saying yes to food for quite a while. Plus, it's a lot easier to cheat when you don't have to worry about divorce or detention hall. On the bright side, you're not alone. A whopping 50 percent of our beach beauties cheat occasionally. Only about 30 percent of them never cheat, while a naughty 20 percent cheat often. None of this should give you an excuse to cheat, but you can relax and know that you are not a failure (and you're not alone!) if you do.

Realistically, you're going to have to suck it up and deal with it. You can stick with this plan. You can also plan to have a little something every once in a while. When we feel the need to go off plan, we plan it. We're still on plan! Get it? We'll never have to beat ourselves up afterward. We planned on that piece of birthday cake; now we're going to eat it and enjoy it, and tomorrow we're back on sugar-free Jell-O. If you do succumb to an unplanned, perhaps naughty cheat, don't fret. You don't have to start over; you didn't undo the progress you made. Just learn from your Krispy Kreme moment, and move forward.

Q: My husband and I eat out frequently and I am trying to get some new ideas. I usually play it safe and stick to salads, but I would like suggestions for eating in regular or chain restaurants. I know that a lot of restaurants have Atkins-friendly meals, which might work, but many are still high in fats and are not suitable for the South Beach diet. I am serious about my weight this time, and I vow to get down to my goal and not give up or slip!

3FC: Many restaurants are now advertising low-carb selections on their menus. Many of these meals may not be wise for South Beachers for two reasons. First, the portions served by most restaurants are sinfully large. Always plan to bring home enough for lunch the next day. You can wipe out most of a day's calorie allowance with one restaurant meal. Second, the ingredients in many low-carb selections are high in saturated fat, because restaurants follow the Atkins approach instead of the South Beach method. Before you dive in, be sure to ask if the meat is a lean cut. Is the skin removed before cooking? Is the dish fried, or cooked in butter?

For smart selections, you can usually find something at a steakhouse. Order grilled chicken with a sweet potato without the butter or sugar, and a salad with light dressing. Shish kebabs are also usually acceptable. If rice is served, make sure it is brown rice. Steer away from pilafs that might have ingredients that aren't allowed, like pasta or high GI vegetables. The vegetable of the day can be good, but check to see if it comes in a vat of butter before ordering. Lastly, there is always the trusty salad. Question the server about the ingredients in the dressing. Most restaurants offer a grilled chicken salad or have a salad bar to enjoy. Okay, salad isn't imaginative, but it works in a pinch.

You can also check out our list of food dos and don'ts that our South Beach beauties have compiled during their stay on the beach.

the golden and rotten egg awards for the best and worst entrées on the beach

Tony Roma's Ribs

Rotten Egg: Ribs! The sauce is too high in sugar.
Golden Egg: Grilled chicken and grilled vegetables.

● *Continued on next page* ●

Boston Market

Rotten Egg: Anything in gravy, which is most of the menu.
Golden Egg: Southwest Grilled Chicken Salad, hold the tortillas.

Ruby Tuesday

Rotten Egg: Most of it. Atkins-approved doesn't mean South Beach–approved.
Golden Egg: White Chicken Chili for a low-carb, low-fat meal.

Chicks' Tip: Kudos to Ruby Tuesday for including their nutrition information right on the menu. It's horrifying, but good education (or entertainment, depending on how you look at it) while you wait for your meal.

Red Lobster

Rotten Egg: Anything fried or broiled, and also the biscuits.
Golden Egg: Crab legs, grilled fish. Veggies, hold the butter.

Lonestar Steakhouse

Rotten Egg: The Cajun Ribeye, with over 1,000 calories and 100g of fat!
Golden Egg: Sweet Bourbon Salmon, steamed veggies, and black bean soup.

Golden Corral

Rotten Egg: Everything but the green beans and lettuce.
Golden Egg: Green beans and lettuce.

Wendy's

Rotten Egg: The sandwiches.
Golden Egg: Chili, Spring Mix Salad, and a reduced-fat dressing.

Outback

Rotten Egg: BBQ'd anything, potatoes, and rice.
Golden Egg: Chicken on the Barbie, hold the sauce, and veggies, no butter.

Chicks' Tip: While the Web site www.outback.com doesn't provide nutritional data, it is full of tips on how to order your meals for special needs. Three cheers for their cooperation!

south beach diet in an eggshell

Professional Counseling No. However, if you subscribe to the official South Beach diet Web site, you can post nutrition questions for their dietitians to answer.

Support System No meetings, but there are a lot of South Beach support forums on the Internet, including our own Fat Chicks on the Beach group at www.3fatchicks.com.

Fitness Factor Barely there. Dr. Agatston suggests exercise but doesn't require it. Other than the two pages in the book of reasons why exercise is good for you, you're on your own.

Family-Friendly Very! Once you hit Phase 2, you can feed your family on the same healthy foods you will enjoy.

Pros It's very heart healthy, provides energy, and is easy to follow.

● *Continued on next page* ●

Cons Forbidden food list can make it harder to stick to. You need more time to plan meals.

$$ Can be initially more expensive, because you are restocking your pantry with new foods, but it evens out over time.

The Person This Diet Is Best For Someone who likes a very structured diet, doesn't mind eating from a limited list of foods, and may be interested in improving her heart health.

recipes from the front lines

Eggs don't have to be just scrambled or sunny-side up. Here are a couple of recipes that practically let you forget about those white oval things in the ingredients list!

When you really need a dose of good ol' breakfast food, try this "French toast." It might not be made with thick slices of bread, but it's extra tasty with turkey bacon and coffee!

mock french toast

4 egg whites
1 egg
1 teaspoon vanilla
¼ cup ricotta cheese
Dash cinnamon
1 packet of granular sugar substitute
Butter spray
Sugar-free maple syrup

Mix everything but the butter spray and the syrup in a bowl. Pour into pan on medium heat just like you are making pancakes. Top with butter spray and syrup and *enjoy!*

This is a standard recipe in the South Beach book, but many of our members were not pleased with the flavor. We created our own version, which is a variation of a family recipe we've eaten for many years. These mini quiches are perfect for breakfast, snacks, or even as a side dish. They freeze well, so you can prepare them in advance. Just thaw them and zap them in the microwave for a few seconds to serve.

anytime spinach quiche cups to go

Two 10-ounce packages of frozen chopped spinach, thawed
  and squeezed dry
1½ cups egg substitute, equal to 6 eggs
1½ cups nonfat cottage cheese
¼ teaspoon salt
Freshly cracked black pepper to taste
4 tablespoons freshly grated Parmesan cheese

Preheat oven to 375°F. Spray a 12-cup muffin pan with nonstick cooking spray. Combine all ingredients except Parmesan cheese. Divide among muffin cups and bake for 20 minutes. Sprinkle each cup with 1 teaspoon of Parmesan cheese and return to oven. Continue to bake 10 minutes more, or until firm and lightly browned. Loosen cups with a narrow spatula and remove to plate to serve. If preparing in advance, remove to wire rack to cool, then refrigerate or freeze as desired.

This is a sweeter variety of chili, suitable for all phases of the South Beach diet. If dried chipotle pepper is unavailable, you may substitute your favorite chili powder. If you are in Phase 2 or 3, you may serve the chili with low-fat sour cream and shredded reduced-fat cheddar cheese. Are you drooling yet?

vegetarian chili

Serves 4 generously

2 tablespoons olive oil
1 large sweet onion, chopped
2 red bell peppers, seeded and chopped
4 cloves garlic, minced
1 cup canned vegetable broth
32-ounce can crushed tomatoes
14-ounce can black beans, drained
14-ounce can kidney beans, drained
Freshly cracked black pepper to taste
1 to 2 teaspoons dried chipotle pepper powder, or to taste

Over moderate heat, add olive oil to a stockpot or Dutch oven. Add onion, peppers, and garlic and sauté for 3 to 5 minutes, or until soft. Stir in ½ cup of the vegetable broth, and the crushed tomatoes. Add beans to mixture and combine well. If too thick, add additional vegetable broth, up to ½ cup more. Gradually season with chipotle pepper, to taste. Reduce heat and simmer 10 to 20 minutes, stirring occasionally.

When you're about to pull into your local diner's parking lot for a bacon cheeseburger deluxe, try driving home instead to make this delicious salad. It has everything your body is craving—except the bun and extra calories!

bacon cheeseburger salad

Serves 1

FOR THE SALAD:

6 ounces 95% lean ground beef, cooked and crumbled

2 slices turkey bacon, cooked and crumbled

4 cups salad greens

1 cup diced tomato

½ cup chopped dill pickle

6 tablespoons chopped red onion

½ cup reduced-fat cheddar cheese

FOR THE TOMATO VINAIGRETTE:

½ cup chopped tomatoes

2 tablespoons white wine vinegar

½ teaspoon dried basil

½ teaspoon dried thyme

¼ teaspoon ground mustard

Pinch coarse black pepper

½ packet Splenda or other sweetener

Combine Tomato Vinaigrette ingredients in a blender and pulse for a few seconds until combined; set aside.

Combine salad ingredients in a bowl. Add vinaigrette and toss well.

Per serving: 282 calories, 12 grams fat, 16 grams carbs, 5 grams fiber, 29 grams protein

Words to Live By

My weakness has always been food and men—in that order.
—DOLLY PARTON

Never eat more than you can lift. —MISS PIGGY

low-carb chicks
the atkins diet

ONE OF THE BIGGEST dieting trends to take American waist-lines by storm in recent history is the carb cutting approach to weight loss. For all of you who are still eating your burgers on a bun, carb-limiting diets are radical programs that let you eat all the bacon and eggs you can fry up in a pan, but won't let you get any-where near a biscuit. Carb-cutting plans have always been a challenge for us Dixie chicks because they eliminate most of the staples of south-ern cooking, like cornbread, sweet potato pie, hush puppies, and yes, much to our horror, even pecan pie!

Now, we aren't nutritionists, but we understand enough about food to know that any diet that doesn't let you eat biscuits and gravy with your bacon and eggs can't be too balanced. The mere thought of starting on a low-carb diet is enough to make the Colonel himself roll over in his Kentucky grave.

The low-carb approach does have some definite advantages, how-ever. Like bacon, for example—and chicken wings. The Atkins plan, which is king of the low-carb diets, lets you eat juicy steaks dripping in herb butter, roasted chicken complete with crispy skin, and omelets stuffed with cheddar cheese, which is probably one of the reasons why so many of us put this plan on our personal weight-loss throne. Who could get hungry or be tempted to cheat when your diet buffet includes all that delicious fat? But hang on to your tenderloins, because there's a catch. While it's true that you can have unlimited protein and fat, you should only eat them in moderation, and you can never eat a burger on a bun.

Wait a minute, did we say moderation? Yes, we did. We realize that's a word that many people don't realize is associated with the Atkins diet, but we're here to tell you moderation matters, even when you're dining with Dr. Atkins.

Sadly for all of us fat chicks in search of the diet rainbow, the Atkins plan isn't the steak and cheese free-for-all that it appears to be. There are portion restrictions. And while there are now lots of your favorite trigger foods at your local grocery store marked with the scarlet A, meaning Atkins-approved, those low-carb treats, although exciting and satisfying in theory, can go over like a lead balloon when what you're really craving is a double chocolate brownie or a super-sized order of fries. In fact, the first time we tasted a rich, chocolaty low-carb brownie, we had childhood flashbacks to the time our big brother talked us into eating dirt by telling us it tasted like chocolate. So just be prepared; there are going to be moments of temptation, even on Atkins, when no approved substitutes will do, and your willpower will have to prevail over your sweet tooth.

The Atkins plan is divided into four phases. The beginning phase, Induction, covers the first two weeks of the plan. This, as any chick who has ever cut carbs will tell you, is when you come face-to-face with the beast—the dreaded carb cravings!

Induction is a lot like diet boot camp and you can bet dollars to doughnuts that it will *not* be a cakewalk! But the good news is that many chicks see drastic weight loss during this initial phase. Dropping a few pounds sure does make it easier to just say no, even when you want a french fry so bad you would eat a birthday candle if it was dipped in ketchup. In fact, many low-carb chicks are so happy with the rapid results during Induction that they are reluctant to move on to the second phase, which is called Ongoing Weight Loss (OWL), hoping to become supermodel slim in record time.

Ready for the next fly in the ointment? Because you know there is one. While it is true that there is usually a hefty weight loss in this early phase, what you're losing is mostly water, and you can only lose so much water weight before you have to level out and move on to the more measured OWL phase of the diet, where results are less rapid and romantic but more sensible and sustainable. If you have a lot of weight to lose, Atkins says you can stay on Induction for up to six months. Lighter low-carb chicks, however, are encouraged to move on to the next phase after the first two weeks.

During Induction you are only allowed twenty carbs per day. For nondieting chicks, twenty carbs is equal to half of a Moon Pie or a six-ounce Coke. Kind of depressing to think about that, isn't it? I mean, who can eat *half* of a Moon Pie? And how many ounces of Coke are in a Big Gulp anyway? But there is some good news. While you can't polish off that Moon Pie and chase it with a Yoo-Hoo, you can eat four cups of vegetables, a few ounces of select cheese, and virtually unlimited amounts of meat and butter—all for twenty carbs. Starting to feel a little better about a low-carb future now? We neither. So let's sweeten the pot a little, because there are a few irresistible elements of a carb-cutting plan that have led fat chicks to just say no to white bread for nearly three decades and counting.

The goal during Induction is to achieve a physical state called *ketosis.* Ketosis is a condition in which you are burning your fat stores, using them as fuel rather than holding on to them in your hips for that rainy day that never comes. This gives a whole new meaning to the phrase "running on empty," doesn't it? When you restrict your carbs, you trick your body into using your stored fat as energy. This triggers a release of those magical *ketones* (substances released when the body breaks down fat for energy), which are then released as waste products into your urine. We know, this doesn't sound too ladylike, but if you think about the fact that in ketosis you are literally whizzing away your fat stores, you can really start to appreciate this brand of bio-chemistry. And if you think this sounds like a dream come true, just wait!

On Atkins, you can have almost any kind of meat you want, even a double cheeseburger with the works (except, of course, the bun and the fries), with very few limits on quantity. You also can eat lots of veggies. Of course, you can't just eat any old thing that grows in the garden. Corn is a definite no-no, as are potatoes and other starchy vegetables. There is, however, a long list of other vegetables to choose from. You can get the full list in the Atkins book, or visit www.3fatchicks.com/atkins for recent updates.

We don't want to kid you, though. Carb-cutting plans are not easy, quick-fix diets. No matter which way you slice the white bread, Induction is difficult. Even though carb-cutting diets let you eat a lot of foods that are taboo on most other plans, you can only eat so many buttered steak and salad dinners before you start to miss the bread and baked potatoes. And a cheeseburger can never really become deluxe without fries and a sesame seed bun. As enticing as the selections are on Atkins, the approved food list is short, and we low-carb chicks with a taste for culinary adventure do tend to get a little bored. If you can stick it out through Induction though, the next phase will allow the addition of more choices, so hang on to your lamb chops and put down those dinner rolls!

In the Ongoing Weight Loss phase of the Atkins plan, you will begin to gradually add carbs back into your life, so you'll have more fun creating your menus. Don't get too excited; by gradually, we mean you'll be adding carbs at a snail's pace of five per day, raised on a weekly basis. This may seem painfully slow, but then again, in the world of weight loss, good things come to those who are willing to wait.

On the Atkins plan, you are almost guaranteed to lose weight if you stick to the food list. Why? Because, frankly, there isn't anything on the food list that we love to pig out on. We know we're not going to gorge on boiled eggs and pork chops for a midnight snack. And a hunk of cream cheese on a spoon just isn't the same as a nice big slice of cheesecake.

As long as you stay in ketosis, you can keep adding more carbs each week. You are able to measure whether you are in ketosis with special ketone test strips that you can find at your local pharmacy. Due to some unfortunate side effects of ketosis—bad breath, for example—not all chicks choose the ketosis route, even though this is how the plan is written. If you are unsure about ketosis, a quick trip to your doctor should help you make the decision. In any case, as long as you are losing weight, you can add nuts, berries, and of course, *more vegetables* to your diet.

As you near your goal weight, you need to put the brakes on and get ready for lifetime maintenance. The name for this phase is Pre-Maintenance. In this phase, you can add a little more variety while you add more carbs to your diet. The idea is to slow down your weight loss and begin to massage the program from a crash diet into a lifestyle.

The final phase of the Atkins plan is called Maintenance. In this phase, now that you have discovered a goal weight that you can maintain comfortably and consistently, you learn to eat so that you can stay just the way you are. If you start to gain or slip back into old eating habits, it is suggested that you start Induction again. Now there's some incentive to stay on plan!

The most common problem that chicks encountered on this plan was, obviously, the carb cravings. A huge chunk of some of the world's most delicious foods are forbidden to us on this plan, and you never get to dip anything in syrup, so how could we not start to experience a few cravings? And it can be very depressing to contemplate living the rest of your life without eating at least a hush puppy or two. Our chicks tell us that the carb cravings were the most severe during Induction, where the Atkins camp refers to a single bite of illegal food as "the taste of failure."

The rigid structure and food restrictions, however, also helped a lot of our low-carb chicks. If they managed to do without those periodic nibbles of forbidden fruit, many were able to get past their carb cravings entirely. Atkins also encourages portion control, because let's face it, it's just easier to say no to a third meatball than another helping of peach cobbler.

Among the low-carb chicks who quit the Atkins plan, most said the lack of choices made them want carbs even more, and they feared bingeing. And as we are three chicks who have been known to eat a four-course meal off a dessert cart, we certainly understand. The Pre-Maintenance and Maintenance phases allow more carbs, but many chicks never make it that far.

But what about the low-carb chicks who reach their goal weight? One very common mistake we chicks make is to think that we can go back to our old way of eating once the diet is over, so we make a bee-line for the nearest bakery once we're finally free. Low-carb chicks have it especially hard because they didn't lose weight by just cutting back portions of their standard fare. Having eliminated entire groups of food from their diet, they often end up feeling like they deserve a reward for all the deprivation—a reward that often involves a carb-athon filled with cake, fritters, and fluffy biscuits.

Can you stick with the Atkins plan for the rest of your life? Studies show that low-carb diets promote rapid weight loss initially, more than low-fat diets offer. These same studies also show, however, that low-carb dieters regain their weight faster than low-fat dieters. A study based on records kept by the National Weight Control Registry showed that not many low-carb dieters were able to maintain their weight loss by continuing a low-carb lifestyle, because in the end, as many fat and formerly fat chicks feel, life without starch is no life at all. Those chicks who increased carbs and reduced fat during Maintenance, and adopted a program that looks more like the South Beach plan, stood a better chance of keeping the weight off permanently.

If you're considering a carb-cutting plan, here are some of the questions and answers from our low-carb chicks about what life is really like in the land of no flour or sugar.

meet the atkins chicks

Debra from Illinois

I'm a forty-six-year-old credit support coordinator. I'm divorced with two daughters and a son, and my seventeen-year-old daughter is low-carbing with me. My parents are both diabetic and I'm hoping the Atkins diet will help me avoid that problem in my life. I lost thirty pounds once before on Atkins but picked the weight back up. This time, though, I have my daughter doing the plan with me, we're supporting each other, plus I have the support of my friends at work and at 3FC, which makes all the difference!

Rosie from New Jersey

I need strict rules when it comes to dieting. For me, it's all or nothing. Atkins helps me feel in complete control, especially where trigger foods are concerned. I am eating very healthy, more fish and veggies and I am taking vitamins. I am taking care of myself for once!

Kim from New Jersey

My biggest problem in losing weight has been the biggest problem in my life: I do not know or understand the word moderation. I'm either all or not at all. And when I put all my effort into something, then other things have to give. So now that I am on Atkins and really trying to follow the program, my house is a mess! I've tasted pretty much everything in my lifetime. Now I need to again taste the feeling of being thin and active with my family. I am finding Atkins really works well with my lifestyle. I just need to keep reminding myself that I have a different metabolism than my husband and children and can't eat like they do. But when I am sixty my family will hopefully care less that I ate differently than they did, especially if they can look back on the bike rides we took together.

Q: I would trade my right arm for a loaf of bread right now! I thought this diet was supposed to take away my carb cravings. Isn't there anything I can do?

3FC: All you can do is hang in there, baby! It may sound cliché, but that doesn't make it any less true. The Atkins Induction phase is based on the theory that your blood sugar needs to be stabilized in order to cut the carb cravings. If you've only been on Atkins a short time, it may take you a few more days to get past this. You may not be past the cravings until the end of this first two-week phase. So stick with it, and if you don't cheat at all, you'll have fewer cravings and the hard part will be over sooner rather than later, we promise! Nibbles of carbish foods can set you back, so it's important to fill up on protein and fats right now. Try snacking on foods like string cheese and nuts to help cut the craving, or eat smaller but more frequent meals.

The book *Atkins Essentials* says that if you haven't overcome your carb cravings by the end of Induction, you are either cheating or refusing to let go. We can buy the part about cheating—maybe you have eaten some hidden carbs that you didn't realize weren't allowed on Induction—but refusal to let go should be reserved for death or *Oprah* tickets. If you're still craving carbs, it isn't a craving, it is true love. If you're a chick who loves carbs and just can't live without them after two weeks of struggling, maybe you should just mosey on over to another chapter and see what some of the less carb-restrictive diets have to offer. This is a diet, not a chamber of horrors. It's important to remember that and find a way to lose weight that you can enjoy and that you are able to maintain long-term.

Q: Whenever I tell someone I'm following Atkins, they cringe and warn me that it's dangerous to my health. I try to explain that the studies say this is a safe diet, but they won't listen. Do I have to go through the rest of my life defending my diet?

3FC: Just the term *low-carb*, and more specifically *Atkins diet*, can elicit the same disapproving looks that are usually reserved for adultery, embezzlement, or a second slice of chocolate cheesecake. To be frank, we don't know if your friends are right or wrong. There really aren't any studies that show this type of diet to be safe long-term. The only studies that have been conducted so far lasted six months to a year. The Atkins plan and other low-carb diets have been around for a long time, but no one has been keeping score. Sure, they are effective for weight loss, but we don't know if they will increase your chances of heart disease or create other problems down the road.

Beef, for example, is a staple of the average low-carb diet, but recent studies have shown that regular meat consumption can significantly increase the risk of colon cancer. Low-carb diets are higher in fat and usually include high percentages of saturated animal fats. Studies from Cambridge University and from the *Journal of the National Cancer Institute* report that the rate of breast cancer among premenopausal women who ate the most animal fat was one-third higher than that of women who ate the least animal fat. If you are eating more of these products, then it stands to reason that you are increasing your chances of disease later on. The Atkins Foundation offers dissenting opinions about common low-carb concerns on their Web site, but they sound like they were written by a PR rep rather than a doctor. We recommend that you discuss any concerns with your physician and have regular physical exams to make sure you stay healthy.

It may be years before we really know the long-term effects of low-carb dieting. In the meantime, stick to your diet if you feel comfortable with it. Losing weight will certainly improve your health, and a low-carb diet is still a healthier option than staying fat. The next time your friends offer advice, just let them know that you are aware of the health concerns but comfortable with your choices.

Q: I've considered going on a low-carb plan, but I just don't get it. How can you eat all that fatty food and still lose weight?

3FC: That is really a very common question, and it's one that even we still wonder about a little. But the bottom line is, when we tried low-carb dieting, it really did work! Low-carb dieting isn't just butter and bacon. You can eat lean meats, seafood, salads, and plenty of vegetables. And of course, you are allowed cream, cheese, sausages, and other fatty foods, but you can eat or not eat as much saturated fat as you choose. Many experts believe low-carb dieting works because you are actually eating less than you were when you were not dieting. Since your food choices are limited, you don't have as many foods to choose from, so you eat less. Also, the protein you are eating helps keep you full longer. It takes longer to digest, so you don't get the munchies like you do when eating packages of nonfat cookies, for example. You usually end up eating less than you think. If you really can't say good-bye to bread, pick another reduced-calorie plan. The main thing is that you pick a diet you can live with.

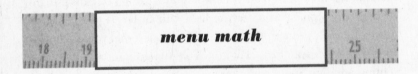

menu math

Why does cutting back on carbs help us lose weight? The answer is not magical properties in fat and protein that get us skinny, it's fewer calories. High-carb foods are often more calorie dense than the same portion of a lower-carb fruit or vegetable.

Here are some comparisons:

1 cup white, long-grain rice: 205 calories
1 cup steamed broccoli: 52 calories

1 medium baked russet potato: 168 calories
1 cup green beans: 44 calories

1 English muffin: 133 calories
1 cup sliced strawberries: 52 calories

1 hamburger bun: 120 calories
2 cups sliced cucumber: 16 calories

1 cup spaghetti: 197 calories
1 cup spaghetti squash: 42 calories

STRUTTING OUR STUFF

I followed the Induction guidelines from www.atkins.com and tried to stick to the plan as closely as possible. I chose foods from the list that I enjoyed and didn't think about the calories at all. At the end of each day, I nervously logged my daily food and assumed I'd eaten over 2,000 calories' worth of fatty foods. I was shocked to see that my average was 1,100 to 1,300 calories each day! Regardless of the lack of carbs, I was still just on another low-calorie diet. I lost about two pounds per week. I couldn't stick to the plan, though, because I thought it was too limited and I didn't think it was healthy enough for me, personally. I don't have any health issues that require me to limit carbs, and my weight is affected more by the calories I consume, and by exercise. —SUZANNE 3FC

Q: I just started on Atkins and I'm going to a covered dish dinner. What can I take that I am allowed to eat, that doesn't scream, "Look at me; I'm on a low-carb diet!"

3FC: We live in the South, so every potluck dinner we've ever attended involves a parade of covered dishes, all of which include some combination of rice, cream of mushroom soup, or Ritz crackers. While that would make any Junior League president proud, it doesn't do much for us Atkins chicks, and it can make our own carb-free contributions to the table very unpopular at supper. After all, what nondieter would ever pass up potato chip casserole in favor of crudités? With the proper covered dish accessories, however, you can make the tastiest dish on the table, without blowing your cover.

Low-Carb Tips for Uncertain Chicks

- Vegetables don't have to be drenched with carb-laden sauces to taste good. They can be seasoned with bacon or butter, or you can try adding olive oil and a few simple herbs or spices. Buy fresh or frozen vegetables for the best flavor.
- For crunch, you can add slivered almonds instead of corn flakes or crackers.
- Try topping your casseroles with shredded or grated Parmesan cheese. You can make nearly any vegetable into a tasty casserole by using heavy cream in place of creamy soups. See our Carbless Cauliflower Gratin on page 68.

Q: What do the shades of Ketostix mean? This morning I was deep purple, but I ate a breath mint and now I'm only light purple.

3FC: It's unlikely that your breath mint changed your test strip. Regardless, don't live by the stick. If you are in ketosis, that is good enough. The most popular theory is that color changes with hydration. Drinking extra water can lighten the shade, just as lack of water can make it darker; however, that isn't the only reason the color may change.

The shades of the pad can also change depending on factors such as foods you have recently eaten, your metabolism, recent exercise, medications, or various other medical conditions. A darker shade of purple doesn't necessarily mean you've become more of a fat-burning machine. Continue to test your stick at the same time each day. If you are losing weight, don't worry about it.

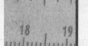

clipped wings: ketosis

Those who say you can attract more flies with honey than vinegar obviously have never been in ketosis. Pickled breath isn't your only concern. Other side effects of ketosis can include nausea, weakness, dehydration, fatigue, insomnia, and headaches. As daunting as this may sound, there are a few things you can do to ease the symptoms.

- Drink water, water, and more water!
- For nausea, try diet ginger ale.
- Get a full night's sleep on a regular basis.
- Exercise every day, even if it's only lightly.
- Chew parsley, sugar-free gum, or mints.
- Eat small meals frequently, even if you aren't hungry.
- Don't cut out caffeine all at once.
- Eat all of your available carbs each day.
- Don't be afraid of fat! Higher fat content will keep you satisfied.

Q: I'm not sure I'm getting the right amount of carbs. I'm careful, but I'm not losing weight. I'm confused about total carbs, hidden carbs, net carbs, and Net Atkins Count.

3FC: Nutrition labeling can be confusing, particularly when it comes to carbohydrates. It is possible that you are consuming more carbs and calories than you really need. The Atkins plan tracks net carbs and Net Atkins Count. Net Atkins Count, listed on Atkins products, refers to a patented clinical method that measures the average blood sugar response to individual products. If a product doesn't list a Net Atkins Count, you will have to determine the net carbs of the product. Deduct the grams of fiber from the total carbohydrates, and this will give you the net carbs. If the glycerin and sugar alcohol counts are also on the nutrition label, you can deduct those too. For whole foods and recipes, just consider total carbs minus fiber. To further confuse things, some manufacturers list "net impact carbs" or "effective carbs." Be sure to read the labeling to see exactly what their definition means, as it can vary.

Be aware also that there may be hidden carbs in your food. These could include fillers in deli meats, powdered mixes, the base for artificial sweeteners, or even alcohol. To be safe, choose the freshest whole ingredients that you can, and always read the labels. Cold cuts and packaged seafood could contain sugars as well as starches for texture and preservative purposes. Also try to limit low-carb convenience foods to occasional use, because they may contain excess calories.

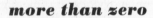

more than zero

Why are there portion limits on zero-carb foods? Well, because in the world of food labels, zero doesn't always mean zero. For example, heavy cream has less than 1 carb per tablespoon serving, so the label says 0 carbs. However, two tablespoons contain 1.2 carbs, four tablespoons contain almost 3 carbs, and a pint of cream has 13 carbs! Coffee also has a little more than one carb per cup. Eggs are approximately .5 carb each, and cheese also has .5 to 1 carb per ounce, depending on what type you're eating. Easily, your zero-carb breakfast can have 8 to 10 carbs. To be safe, use a good nutrition software program to see what your true carb counts are, or follow the guidelines and limit these foods.

Q: I've been on Atkins for three weeks and I'm exhausted. With all the protein I eat, shouldn't I have more energy?

3FC: Carbohydrates are the body's main source of quick energy. Protein is converted to energy, but at a much slower pace than carbs. Are you getting enough carbs? It's easy to think that if dropping to twenty carbs is good, dropping to ten is even better, but this isn't actually the case. As carbs are our chief source of quick energy, you need at least twenty carbs a day to function effectively. Double-check your total carb intake and make sure you are getting at least twenty carbs if you are on Induction, or more if you have graduated to OWL. Also, don't eat all of your carbs in one meal. Try spreading those twenty carbs throughout your day. If you exercise a lot, you may even need to increase your carbs just a little. Try taking a multivitamin, and make sure you drink enough water. If you still don't see an improvement, see your physician, in case there is an underlying problem you don't know about.

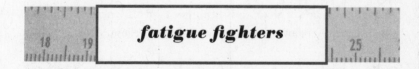

fatigue fighters

- French fries and mashed potatoes aren't the only starch villains to avoid. The couch potato can also foil your dieting efforts. Just sitting around, at the office or at home or in front of

• *Continued on next page* •

the tube, can leave you feeling lethargic. Now, more than ever, you need to get up and move in order to revitalize yourself!

- Make sure that you're hydrated. Dr. Atkins tells us that even slight dehydration can cause fatigue, so drink up!
- Take a tip from kitty and enjoy a catnap. A short nap can be refreshing and make a huge difference in your energy levels for the rest of your day.
- Try a little afternoon delight to rev your engines. Sex gets the blood flowing and your motor humming!

Q: I only eat low-carb versions of everything. I've not had a full-carb candy bar, snack chip, or sandwich in ages! So if I'm only eating low-carb foods, why aren't I losing weight?

3FC: Many experts believe that low-carb diets work because you eliminate entire groups of food and so end up eating fewer calories. Low-carb plans have become so popular that manufacturers are competing for our business. Instead of doing without pasta and candy, we are eating low-carb versions of pasta and candy, and ice cream, snack chips, cakes, and just about anything else you can imagine. The trouble is that we're replacing the calories, and then some. Low-carb diets are like any other diet: you have to eat less than you burn for fuel, and moderation is essential. Try counting your carbs, curbing your snacks, and eating more vegetables or other healthy foods. Pay attention to your list of ingredients. A snack of almonds is healthier than an "energy" bar with a long list of preservatives, high-calorie fillers, and chemicals.

Q: I'm so tired of the same thing for breakfast, what else can I eat? And please don't say bacon and eggs!

3FC: We've seen some really disgusting recipes for pancakes made out of pork rinds, so we feel your pain. We think pork rinds were made for beer and ballgames, not for sugar-free syrup! We have a few alternative palate-pleasing, nontraditional breakfast ideas.

Try making hash browns using shredded zucchini instead of potatoes. Pair them with sausage for a nice change of pace. You can also try
grilling a steak or other juicy meat and top with avocados, or eat leftovers from the night before. Variety is the spice of life, after all, so
what's wrong with eating a little dinner for breakfast?

Another interesting idea we've come across is the infamous breakfast burrito. Use a low-carb tortilla, and fill with any combination of
cheese, sausage, chopped cilantro, tomato, mushrooms, hamburger,
and even bacon and eggs! Or if low-carb bread fits in with your daily
carb count, toast a slice and spread with peanut butter or cream
cheese and a pinch of cinnamon. In the middle of a carb craving, it'll
taste as good as a Reese's cup, we guarantee. If you're really in a
pinch, you can keep ready-to-drink low-carb shakes in the fridge, or
have meal replacement bars handy. They aren't the best choice, but
it's better than going to the Waffle House.

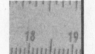

foods that fool your taste buds

We know how difficult it can be to give up your favorite high-
carb foods, but there are substitutes, such as our Chocolate Almonds Diablo on page 69, that can fool your taste buds and
give you an artificial and completely legal carb rush that's almost as good as the one you get after biscuits and gravy on Sunday morning. Well, almost as good anyway. Here are a few ideas
from our Atkins chicks.

● I had the hardest time giving up potatoes and rice, until I
discovered how versatile cauliflower was. Cooked, chopped

● Continued on next page ●

cauliflower is great for a potato salad substitute. Cut raw cauliflower into small, rice-sized pieces, then place in a covered bowl and microwave for a few minutes. It will be mild and just like rice!

• Baking mixes are still wildly expensive and, to be honest, not all that good. If you don't mind the taste of soy flour, you're in luck! Otherwise, try nut flours. Nut flours lose something in texture but gain in taste. New low-carb tortillas and breads on the market are good.

• My downfall has always been pizza. Most low-carb pizza crusts are like disks of flavorless cardboard. I solved my problem by topping low-carb tortillas with pizza toppings and making wraps. I get all of the flavor and the good stuff without having to mentally get past the cardboard barrier.

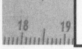

alternachick tips

If you think going low-carb is impossible without including steak, you may be surprised to learn that many vegetarians are also losing weight by following Atkins or other low-carb plans. A few of our vegetarian alternachicks shared their low-carb experiences.

I am a strict vegetarian (not vegan) and am still following the Atkins plan. It was hard at first, but each day I find something that makes it easier. I will never stop being a vegetarian, but I have to get this weight off, so I am in for the long haul. My carb cravings have virtually disappeared, and I am rarely hungry, so that is great. After the first few days, I realized that for every meat product on the plan, there is a vege-tarian substitute, and they usually have low-carb contents as long as they are not breaded. —CHRISTY

I've come to realize that my low-carb diet will never be as low-carb as everyone else's. Most meat substitutes have some carbs, so it's impossible to go very low and still get enough protein. I still feel so much better than when I was on a high-carb diet, and I'm still losing weight. —JANET

I've tried the vegetarian versions of a few low-carb plans. I started on Atkins, then I switched to Carbohydrate Addicts LP, but then I moved on to Protein Power. I think PP is very vegetarian friendly! —CELIA

I tried to do a vegetarian version of Atkins, but it wasn't easy. I spent more carbs on protein products such as tofu or beans and had to cut back on other veggie carbs to make up for it. Since I lost some of my veg-gies, I added a multivitamin daily. I was never able to get a proper bal-ance and eventually realized there was no such thing as a vegetarian Atkins diet. —SHELLY

Q: I was drawn to the Atkins plan because of all the meat, cheese, and eggs, but now I find out I have to eat at least four cups of veggies each day. Even my mother couldn't get me to eat my vegetables. I can manage an occasional salad, but anything beyond that is out of the question!

3FC: You might have come into this diet singing your own personal ren-dition of "Cheeseburger in Paradise," but your mother was right! It is im-portant to get the fiber and nutrients that vegetables offer, even on a high-protein, high-fat diet. So if you don't like plain old vegetables, do what we do, and dress them up a little. Try our Blue Cheese and Pecan Green Beans recipe on page 71; after all, vegetables can be as bland or as extravagant as you like. And particularly when it comes to cauliflower and broccoli, don't forget the power of cheese! Sprinkle everything with a good cheese and you'll be guaranteed to clean your plate. Grilling vegetables will bring out rich, sweet flavors that will surprise you and leave you craving more. Fill a low-carb tortilla with grilled veggies and cheese for a delicious wrap sandwich. Try a vegetable and beef shish kebab for a change of pace! A little imagination can make vegetables irresistible.

And you need them. Vegetables may be your only good source of fiber while on a low-carb diet. They will help keep you regular, especially important since constipation is a common problem among low-carbers. You'll also benefit from antioxidants, which can protect you from heart disease and certain kinds of cancer.

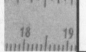

low-carb brown bags

Does your nine to five interfere with your diet? Here are some of the low-carb chicks' best ideas for easy brown bagging the low-carb way. Most of these can be brought to work in an insulated lunch bag.

- peel-and-eat shrimp
- deviled eggs
- homemade soup
- tuna/chicken salad and pork rinds (or Wasa crackers, if your diet permits)
- low-carb yogurt
- antipasto plate
- low-carb wrap rolled with Laughing Cow cheese, ham, and chopped olives
- roast beef rollups with cream cheese and roasted red peppers
- turkey BLT rollups

- veggies and dip
- salad, Caesar or garden
- egg salad on romaine hearts
- leftovers!
- string cheese and nuts

 ## *To Market, to Market*

Shopping for Atkins-friendly foods can seem like a trip to the farm: you have cattle, a chicken coop, a dairy, and a lettuce patch. This means you never have to go into the potato chip barn or down the cookie row. Almost everything you really need in a supermarket can be found in the perimeter of produce, meat, and dairy. This is good news for Atkins chicks in the midst of a chocolate chip attack. If you don't get near it, you can't eat it.

As manufacturers continue to produce low-carb versions of old favorites, we may find the need to explore the inner aisles of breads, sauces, and pastas in search of labels (undoubtedly with large lettering) proclaiming low-carb status. We've trekked through the dark underbelly of carbohydrate-loaded shelves and emerged with our list of Chick Picks for the Atkins On-going Weight Loss stage.

- La Tortilla Factory Low-Carb Tortillas
  www.latortillafactory.com
- LeCarb
- Heinz One Carb Ketchup
  www.heinz.com

● *Continued on next page* ●

- Carbdown Flatout bread
  www.flatoutbread.com
- Atkins Morning Start bars
  www.atkins.com
- Dreamfields pasta
  www.dreamfieldsfoods.com
- Carb Options Asian Teriyaki Sauce
  www.carboptions.com
- Crystal Light Sunrise
  www.crystallight.com
- Hood Carb Countdown milk
  www.hphood.com

Q: Our family has a huge celebration every Fourth of July, complete with grilled burgers, potato salad, and apple pie à la mode. The burger part will be easy—leave off the bun. But how can I resist the potato salad and apple pie? Is it okay to break the diet, just for one day?

3FC: If you can celebrate responsibly, you may be able to go off plan every now and then. Usually, though, you will want to plan ahead and have delicious substitutes available. You have the burger covered; now you just need a side dish and a dessert. Broccoli with cheese sauce is always a hit, even for nondieters. The cheese sauce will also be yummy on the burger!

Nothing hits the spot more on the Fourth of July than a bowl of ice cream. You'll never miss the hot apple pie. Low-carb ice creams are common in every supermarket now, and they're really good! If you want to impress your guests, make our homemade ice cream on page 72 that is so rich and creamy, they'll never believe it's a diet food.

Play hard and get the most out of your holiday. Whether it's a game of touch football or a walk around the block with a loved one, this is one holiday that screams for outdoor activities. Take advantage of it, and forget about the food.

Q: I've been on the Atkins diet for almost three months. I've had a few terrible bouts of constipation, and that isn't like me! What can I do?

3FC: Grab a bottle of Metamucil and repeat after us, "This too shall pass—in twenty-four to forty-eight hours." In the meantime, start working on your water and fiber habits! You should be drinking at least eight 8-ounce glasses of water a day. Stay away from caffeinated beverages. The caffeine can dehydrate your body, making bowel movements slower. Be sure that you are eating your daily allotment of vegetables and fruit, and also try to incorporate nuts into your snacks.

You should also make an effort to fit exercise into your regular schedule. Even a twenty- to thirty-minute daily walk can make a difference in your bowel movements. Don't miss an opportunity to find a bathroom when the urge hits.

beating the low-carb blues

Low-carbohydrate plans made the headlines again in March 2004, when scientists announced that low-carb diets, such as the Atkins program, could cause depression and mood swings. Researchers at MIT, one of the country's top research universities, discovered that high levels of carbs and low levels of proteins were key to producing enough serotonin to regulate our moods. Low-carb dieters frequently complained of depression or irritability but did not realize that their new lifestyle could be the cause. The effects were not always seen in individuals with normal serotonin levels but were noticeable in people who had had previous problems with depression or had bipolar disorder. New

● *Continued on next page* ●

low-carb dieters were surprised by the news, but some seasoned dieters experienced an "aha" moment.

If you have a history of depression or bipolar disease, you may want to reconsider choosing a low-carb diet. If you choose this route and notice any problems, consult your physician. She may decide to prescribe medication used to treat depression. Another option may be to gradually increase your carbs until you feel more comfortable. Exercise is also important for mitigating depression. One hour of aerobic exercise per day will make you feel much better, plus it will burn more calories so you reach your goal faster!

Q: Does anybody notice that her sex life has improved since starting a low-carb diet? I've been on Atkins for two months now, my sex drive has gone through the roof, and I have much stronger orgasms!

3FC: Okay, all of you fellas out there, don't make any mad dashes to Wal-Mart for a gift copy of *The Atkins Diet* for your wives before you read this, because while there are a couple of different reasons why low carbs could lead to better sex, they may not apply to everybody.

First, there is a connection between high blood sugar, or hormonal imbalances aggravated by excess weight, and low sex drive. It is a not-uncommon side effect in diabetics who have a problem controlling their blood sugar. Low sex drive, fatigue, and other unpleasant symptoms can occur. When you are on a low-carb diet, you're regulating your blood sugar much more than before you went on the diet. These symptoms can be improved by the diet, but only if you had the problems with sugar and/or hormones to begin with.

If your blood sugar and hormones are normal, then you could possibly still experience increased sexual appetite while on Atkins because of an increase in self-esteem. If you've been on a diet for two months, you're probably getting more exercise, which also stimulates libido. Losing a few extra pounds can take stress off your body and improve your confidence in how good you look in your birthday suit.

You'll experience this boost with any weight loss, not just the low-carb kind.

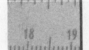

snack on this

If you're aching for some extra snacks but don't want to blow your diet, try a one-carb snack! These snacks have approximately one carb each.

- 2 ounces provolone cheese
- 8 ounces soy milk
- ½ celery stalk with 1 tablespoon of cream cheese
- 1 beef hot dog, no bun
- 6 ounces steamed crab with 2 tablespoons drawn butter
- 2 teaspoons hummus
- 1 deviled egg
- 1 cup peel-and-eat shrimp with 2 tablespoons of tartar sauce
- 1 roasted chicken breast

atkins in an eggshell

Professional Counseling Yes and no. You can call Atkins information agents at a toll-free number if you have questions about

● *Continued on next page* ●

the plan. Don't expect a "You go, girl!" or ribbons. This is just for nitty-gritty diet questions.

Support System There is nothing official from Atkins. You won't attend meetings, but there are countless unofficial Atkins support forums on-line, including at www.3fatchicks.com.

Fitness Factor Atkins encourages exercise throughout the program, but there is no specific exercise plan. Also, according to the American Council on Exercise, "carbohydrates are essential for an effective workout."

Family-Friendly Not very! This plan requires additional cooking for the dieter's special meals if a balanced dinner is to be fed to kids. Most pediatricians recommend that children not follow a low-carb diet.

Pros Quick weight loss, particularly in the beginning. You'll be less hungry than on some diets, as protein suppresses appetite.

Cons Restaurant choices are limited and get boring. Can be difficult to stick to long-term. The jury is still out on long-term safety.

$$ Meat and other staples are costly, and low-carb specialty foods are very expensive.

The Person This Diet Is Best For Someone who loves meat and eggs, who doesn't mind taking the extra time needed to prepare menus, and who doesn't get bored easily.

recipes from the front lines

When you're eating foods that are fat- and protein-heavy, try switching out the beef and butter for more healthful options. Here's one of our own recipes that is low in carbs and includes *good* fats from fish and olive oil.

tilapia with slow-roasted grape tomatoes

Serves 4

1 pint grape tomatoes
2 tablespoons olive oil
½ teaspoon kosher salt
2 tablespoons white wine
1 small shallot, minced (1 tablespoon)
Freshly cracked black pepper to taste
4 tilapia fillets (4 ounces each)
4 tablespoons freshly grated or shaved Parmesan cheese

Preheat oven to 325°F. Toss tomatoes with olive oil and salt in the bottom of a 2-quart shallow casserole dish. Roast in oven, uncovered, for 30 minutes. Remove pan from oven; lightly smash tomatoes with back of wooden spoon, stir in wine, shallots, and black pepper; return to oven for additional 20 minutes. Slow roasting brings out the sweetness in the tomatoes;

• *Continued on next page* •

don't be tempted to skip this step. Remove dish from oven and stir mixture. Increase heat to 400°F. Lay tilapia fillets across tomato mixture and dust with additional black pepper to taste. Return to oven for 12 to 15 minutes or until fish flakes easily with a fork. Remove fish to serving platter and spoon tomato mixture across top. Top with freshly grated or thinly shaved Parmesan and serve.

Per serving: 4 grams total carbs (3 net carbs), 198 calories, 9 grams fat, 2 grams saturated fat, 1 gram fiber, 24 grams protein

---

Here's a cheesy solution that helps our low-carb chicks dance to their own tune, even when everybody around them is doing the mashed potato. This is a very rich and creamy casserole, and it hits the spot when you have a hankering for potatoes.

carbless cauliflower gratin

Serves 4

Nonstick cooking spray
1 bag (16 oz) frozen cauliflower
½ cup chopped onion
¼ teaspoon salt
¼ teaspoon white pepper
1 cup shredded sharp cheddar cheese
¾ cup heavy cream

Preheat oven to 350°F. Spray a 9 × 9-inch pan with cooking spray, and set aside. Thaw cauliflower in a colander under running water. Cut any large florets into bite-sized pieces. Spread cauliflower evenly in pan. Sprinkle onion over cauliflower and season with salt and pepper. Top with the cheddar cheese, then drizzle the cream evenly over the top. Bake for 40 minutes, or until casserole is thick and golden on top.

Per serving: 9 grams total carbs (6 net carbs), 303 calories, 26 grams total fat, 16 grams saturated fat, 3 grams fiber, 10 grams protein

Here's a devilishly sweet solution, guaranteed to fool even the most indulgent sweet tooth without costing you carbs.

chocolate almonds diablo

Serves 8

Butter
3 tablespoons Splenda
1 tablespoon unsweetened cocoa powder
½ teaspoon cinnamon
1 egg white
2 teaspoons heavy cream
1 cup whole almonds

Preheat oven to 300°F. Line a baking sheet with foil and spread with enough butter to coat. Combine Splenda, cocoa, and cinnamon in a small bowl and set aside. Whisk egg white and cream in a small mixing bowl until frothy; stir in almonds. Carefully drain away excess liquid. Add dry ingredients to the almonds and stir to coat. Spread almonds on baking sheet in a

• *Continued on next page* •

single layer. Bake for 15 to 20 minutes, until almonds are toasted and dry. Use a spatula to loosen any almonds that are stuck to foil, then cool on pan. Remove to a storage container and seal tightly.

Per serving: 7 total carbs (5 net carbs), 184 calories, 16 grams total fat, 2 grams saturated fat, 2 grams fiber, 7 grams protein

When you're deep in the trenches trying to wait out a nacho attack, let this recipe for a nacho casserole take you up over the next hill.

when-you-really-need-nachos pie

Serves 4

8 ounces shredded Monterey jack cheese
½ cup cottage cheese
1 cup chunky salsa
5 eggs
½ cup buttermilk
1 tablespoon cilantro
¼ teaspoon salt
Sour cream for garnish

Preheat oven to 350°F. Spray a pie pan with nonstick cooking spray and set aside. Combine cheeses and salsa in a medium bowl. Spread into pie pan. Add eggs and buttermilk to bowl and blend well. Add cilantro and salt. Stir, then pour over the salsa and cheese mixture. Bake approximately 40 minutes or until lightly browned and puffed in center. Garnish with sour cream.

Per serving: 8 total carbs (7 net carbs), 351 calories, 24 grams total fat, 13 grams saturated fat, 1 gram fiber, 27 grams protein

---

Dressed up with champagne mustard, salty blue cheese, and sweet pecans, these green beans have a little something for everyone.

blue cheese and pecan green beans

Serves 4

1 teaspoon champagne mustard (Dijon will work as well)
2 teaspoons red wine vinegar
1 teaspoon chopped fresh chives
1 tablespoon minced shallots (about 1 small shallot)
2 tablespoons olive oil
12 ounces fresh green beans, trimmed and cut in bite-sized pieces
¼ cup blue cheese
½ cup pecans

Fill a medium saucepan with 6 to 8 cups of water. Bring to a boil. Meanwhile, mix mustard, vinegar, chives, shallots, and olive oil together in a small bowl; set aside.

Add the green beans to the boiling water, and cook at a low

● *Continued on next page* ●

boil until just tender, approximately 5 to 6 minutes. Drain beans and immediately rinse with cold water. Don't rinse for too long or the beans will get cold, and nobody likes cold green beans.

Pour the drained beans back into the saucepan. Add the oil mixture to the beans and toss to coat well. Add blue cheese and pecans and toss again. Serve immediately.

Per serving: 9 total carbs (5 net carbs), 201 calories, 18 grams total fat, 4 grams saturated fat, 4 grams fiber, 4 grams protein

---

Celebrate your carb independence this Fourth of July with a homemade ice cream that is so yummy, it will give your non-Atkins friends bowl envy!

apple almost ice cream

Serves 8

1 large egg
3 large egg yolks
¾ cup granulated Splenda
1 teaspoon apple pie spice
Pinch salt
3 cups heavy cream
½ teaspoon vanilla extract
1 tablespoon butter
¼ cup chopped pecans

Whisk egg, egg yolks, Splenda, ¾ teaspoon of the apple pie spice, and salt in a small bowl until well blended. Heat cream in a medium, heavy saucepan over medium-low heat, stirring constantly, until cream begins to bubble around edges and is hot. Carefully spoon a little of the hot cream into the egg mixture, whisking constantly to temper the eggs. Add a little more cream and continue to blend well. Slowly pour egg mixture into the saucepan with remaining cream, whisking thoroughly as you go. Continue to cook and stir until mixture coats the back of a spoon, about 2 or 3 minutes. Remove from heat and stir in vanilla extract. Pour mixture into a medium bowl and cover with plastic. Chill at least 4 hours or overnight.

Meanwhile, preheat oven to 325°F. Melt butter in the bottom of a small baking dish. Add pecans, stir, and then sprinkle with the remaining ¼ teaspoon apple pie spice. Toast mixture in oven for about 30 minutes or until lightly browned. Watch carefully that it does not burn. Transfer mixture to a small bowl and allow to cool until you make the ice cream.

To make ice cream: Pour chilled custard mixture into ice cream freezer and freeze according to manufacturer's directions. Add pecans during last few minutes of freezing process and allow mixture to blend evenly.

Per serving: 6 total carbs (6 net carbs), 386 calories, 39 grams fat, 22 grams saturated fat, 0 grams fiber, 4 grams protein

Words to Live By

Stressed *spelled backwards is* desserts. *Coincidence? I think not!*
—AUTHOR UNKNOWN

I worry about scientists' discovering that lettuce has been fattening all along. —ERMA BOMBECK

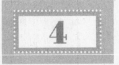

chicks who count
weight watchers

LET'S JUST CUT to the bottom line. Weight Watchers works. Chicks who count on Weight Watchers (WW) do lose weight, and they keep it off too, over the long haul, in greater numbers than any other dieters and all without ever having to say no to a single food group. No wonder Weight Watchers is by far one of the largest, most well-known, and most effective weight-loss programs in the world.

Weight Watchers just plain takes all the fun out of cheating, because you can eat everything that the carbo-loving heart of Dixie has to offer. You can eat fritters, pies, and yes, even those wicked potatoes, but you have to learn to eat them *in moderation*. That word just keeps cropping up everywhere, doesn't it?

Moderation is an unavoidable element in long-term weight loss, and effectively teaching their clients the art of moderation may be what makes Weight Watchers not only the biggest name but also one of the most successful programs of all time. WW teaches moderation as a life skill and gives you tools that you can use for the rest of your life, not just while you are on your way from a size 18 to a size 6.

Weight Watchers weekly meetings are the backbone of the program and almost as easy to find in Anytown USA as a Starbucks. If by some remote chance you live in a town where they don't have a Weight Watchers, you can join Weight Watchers at Home or Weight Watchers Online. These are very good substitutes for the live meetings; however, you won't be experiencing the personal contact, which is really the hallmark of this diet plan.

Some of our chicks squirmed at the thought of going to the meetings but then learned that there's really nothing to be afraid of. We'll admit that before we went to our first meeting, we half expected to find buzzing fluorescent lights with a bunch of metal chairs in a circle, and a couple of sober-looking judges with pens and clipboards standing in front of the dreaded scale just waiting to mortify us—or even worse, hand us a glass of Crystal Light and force us to sweat to the oldies.

When we finally broke down and went to our first Weight Watchers meeting, the reality couldn't have differed more from our fantasies. Weight Watchers meetings are a little like classes, where you learn all about how to lose weight and keep it off, and where you develop the sense of support and community you need to be successful.

Your Weight Watchers community is a crucial part of the program. They will be there for you when you set your goals, celebrate successes, experience setbacks, or trip over stumbling blocks. And almost as important, you will be there for them too. There is no coercion involved with this process. Nobody is forced to participate or contribute, nobody will see how much you weigh, and you won't be forced into circle time, buddy sessions, or any other involuntary socializing.

If going to the meetings just doesn't float your boat, there are other options. WW Online has duplicated almost the entire WW experience on their Web site, located at www.weightwatchers.com. You can join their program for a reasonable monthly fee. You'll have access to weekly topics and to a multitude of user guides and tips, and you can have weekly weigh-ins from the privacy of your own home, which can be a real relief to many of us shy chicks, who are more comfortable stepping on a scale in their private nest than in front of the whole coop.

If you'd like to attend a meeting, but there isn't one near you, then you can join WW at Home. This option is only for people who do not have a meeting in their area. If you subscribe, you will get all of the guidebooks and basic accessories, plus a subscription to *Weight Watchers Magazine*, along with some extra goodies so you can do everything right in your own home. You won't have a regular leader and meeting mates for support, but you will be able to call WW toll-free for six months.

Weight Watchers' latest program theme is called Turn Around, which is not to be confused with our reaction whenever we pass a sweetshop. This kind of turnaround is about turning your life around and starting off in a new and healthier direction. At Weight Watchers there are two paths, or plans, that lead to a total transformation—the big turnaround in your life.

The first is the ever-popular Flex plan. On the Flex plan you count "points" assigned to each food based on calories, fat, and fiber. All foods have a point value. The number of points that you are allowed each day is based on your weight. As you lose weight, your daily targeted number of points will decrease, since you won't need as many calories.

In addition to the daily allotment of points, you'll get more points to use as you choose throughout the week. You can earn up to twenty-eight extra "activity" points each week, just by exercising. Now that's motivation to get moving! You also get another thirty-five points each week to spend as you please, no matter how little you exercise, just because Weight Watchers loves us. If you want to spend a few points each day for small indulgences, that is perfectly fine, or you may enjoy saving them up all week to spend at one big splurge.

The second plan, the Core plan, is Weight Watchers' answer to carb-limited diets. While this isn't a low-carb plan per se, it brings together the most favorable aspects of today's popular low-carb and "good carb" diets, without sacrificing its value as a balanced diet. On Core, your eating is unlimited, as long as you eat Core-approved foods and as long (and here's that pesky moderation idea again) as you eat only until you are no longer hungry.

Like carb-focused plans, the Core plan requires self-control and discipline on our parts, because we're being trusted to understand that "unlimited" does not mean that you can approach every meal like an all-you-can-eat buffet and stuff yourself silly. In other words, we are being trusted to limit ourselves. This isn't always an easy task for us fat chicks, who still insist that the most important part of any balanced meal is seconds. Core, however, is great for chicks who don't want to be bothered with counting points, or who are comfortable with being restricted to a list of permissible foods, rather than being allowed to choose from the whole candy store.

The Core food list is also more liberal than some of the other carb-focused plans out there. You can eat in moderation potatoes (yes, *potatoes*), popcorn, rice, and other starchy foods that are strictly forbidden on other carb-controlled diets, so you actually can get the best of both worlds. But as we all know, you have to give to get, and you will be giving up some of the Flex plan food options—like sugar, alcohol, and juice—on the Core plan. You can eat these non-Core foods, but you have to use the extra weekly point allowance that is given to all members. Or you can use those activity points that you are earning from exercising each day!

Both the Core and the Flex plans give you a lot of freedom, plus extra privileges for extra effort. There's no other mainstream diet on the market today that gives you daily treats for exercising. Regardless of which Weight Watchers plan you're on, you can earn and spend those points any way your pecan-roll-loving heart desires.

All in all, Weight Watchers has the most satisfied and successful group of dieters that we have surveyed at 3fatchicks.com. The majority of dieters who left Weight Watchers did not go to another diet. Instead, they employed the tools they learned at Weight Watchers to limit their own consumption. When they started to pick up weight, they cut back. It's that simple, once you've learned the method. This is strikingly different from the experience of chicks on the wing from other diets: those chicks left diet programs and flew to another coop as fast as their wings could carry them because their old programs had not taught them the arts of moderation and portion control, as Weight Watchers had taught its fledglings. We think that WW succeeds partly because, basically, everything is allowed, as long as you eat *in moderation!*

We talked to our chicks who count about their questions, suggestions, and concerns, about why they thought they were so successful, or why they failed with this plan, and here is a little of what they had to say.

meet the chicks who count

Carol in Tennessee

I began my life skinny, as a one-pound preemie. I stayed underweight until my thirties, when I finally leveled out at a normal weight. When I reached my forties, everything changed and I became overweight. I weighed 176 when I joined Weight Watchers and then lost 33 pounds, though I regained most of it within a few years. I rejoined Weight Watchers with a new commitment and reached my goal of 135 pounds.

I'm sixty-seven years old now, and I've maintained my loss for three years. I walk four miles on my treadmill every morning, and then I plan my points for the day. I couldn't maintain my weight without either one of those routines. I eat well, and the plan is easy to follow. I know that if I continue with the meetings, I will stay at goal. I go to Weight Watchers every week as a Lifetime Member, and I always will.

The Fat Chicks Air In

Carol in Tennessee is our mom, and we are very proud of her for lots of reasons, but most recently, for her renewed commitment to good health, because we want her around forever. We love you, Mom!

• *Continued on next page* •

Dawny from Chesterfield, England

I'm thirty-five years old, married for twelve and a half years, and have a beautiful little three-year-old boy, AJ. I also have two stepdaughters, one of whom has just given us a gorgeous granddaughter, Ella. I have been attending WW meetings since January '04. It was the one New Year's resolution that I actually managed to stick to! I have lost 53½ pounds so far, with only 2 pounds to go to reach my goal weight. I feel that in some ways it has taken for ever and a day, but I know realistically that the weight is more likely to stay off if I lose it slowly. I have come to the conclusion that I will have to be a member of WW for life now, that this is a weight-loss journey that I will have to follow forever. I will always be a fat person, no matter what size the body is. I could so easily go back to how I was before, but I really have no intention of doing that if I can possibly help it. I wish all new Weight Watchers members all the luck in the world. It really does work, you know; you just have to put in a bit of time and effort.

Jill from Canada

One morning fourteen months ago I finally had an epiphany: if I didn't do something soon, I didn't even want to think about what kind of future (if any) was in store for me. Luckily I had a very caring friend who came to that first WW meeting with me. After the meeting I sat in my car and cried. I hadn't weighed myself for so long, and while I knew it would be bad, the number filled me with despair. It seemed insurmountable, but then I thought, "Well, I've got nothing else planned right now and time's going to pass either way. I might as well try this and see what happens." Before I knew it, a month had gone by with noticeable results, so I kept going . . . and going . . . and eventually it just became a way of life. And other benefits came along with the weight loss: if anyone had told me a year ago that I'd be walking, hiking, and playing tennis every week, I wouldn't have believed them. I applied for and got a wonderful new job that I never would have had the confidence to try for a year ago. You know what the very best thing is about losing this weight? Even more than looking better? It's having a feeling of control. For the first time in my life I'm controlling food instead of letting food control me, and that feels better than anything I've ever tasted!

Karen from Ohio

I joined Weight Watchers in the early fall. I lost 59.8 pounds by the beginning of summer and maintained fairly well until my wedding six months later. Then I got too comfortable and gained 11 pounds back. Yuck. *I have since recommitted with renewed vigor to Weight Watchers. You can see the progress in my weight tracker. This new, committed effort is being reinforced by two great friends. One has recommitted as well and the other has made her commitment for the first time. My hubby is a wonderful support and loves the evolving me. I try to keep myself on the Flex plan. I like the bottom line. There's strength for me in numbers.*

Q: I'm having a difficult time working in exercise to earn activity points. Is there any other way to get them?

3FC: In a word, *no!* There is no other way to earn than to burn. Sorry. You have to work in your exercise time. It isn't just about the activity points. You need to exercise to burn fat, build muscle, and strengthen the heart. Exercise should be looked at as a permanent part of your life, like showering, eating, or cleaning. Anything you can consider "aerobic" is exercise. A heavy housecleaning session can even do the trick for beginners if you get your heart rate up. Aim for thirty to sixty minutes a day of exercise. Do it in front of the TV if you must multi-task. If you have a busy, stressful life, you may want to try Pilates or power yoga. They can relax and tone you at the same time. With enough determination, almost anybody can squeeze in a little exercise time. If necessary, start on the weekends and work up to including exercise in your busier workdays. Try to be creative, because regular exercise is as important as moderation in any long-term weight-loss plan.

18 19	25

reality bytes

We all know that exercise will help us lose weight, but sometimes reality just isn't enough to get us out of that recliner and onto the stepper. So the next time you're trying to summon a little motivational lift and thrust, try repeating a few of these reasons to exercise, and reach for the sky.

1. Endorphins are a natural high that last for a long time after you climb off the elliptical machine.
2. Exercise is a great stress reliever. If you're feeling wound up after a rough day at the office, work it out with a little kick-boxing cardio!
3. Muscle takes up less room than fat, so you may drop sizes even if you don't lose weight. Just imagine how great that will feel at your next weigh-in.
4. You'll be more energetic, so you won't have to work as hard to get up off the couch next time, plus the more lean muscle mass you have, the more calories you burn, even when you're lying down.
5. Exercise improves the quality of your sleep, and getting proper rest is not only important to your overall well-being but can also help stave off some extra pounds. Studies have shown that when you're tired, you eat more empty calories and store more fat.
6. You'll have less chance of acquiring certain illnesses, such as arthritis, osteoporosis, and some types of cancer.
7. Exercise is a great cure for the blues and may lessen the symptoms of depression or anxiety.
8. Exercise reduces your "bad" cholesterol level.

9. There's nothing like earning a few activity points to make you feel really good about yourself.
10. When you feel fit and toned, you just feel sexier.

---

i can't believe i ate the whole thing, and other weigh-in nightmares

I was buying refreshments for my son's birthday slumber party. I had bags of chips, a few two-liter bottles of soda, frozen pizzas, cookies, candy bars, and even a box of doughnuts for their breakfast. After I put everything on the belt, I looked up at the person in line behind me, and it was my Weight Watchers leader. —TONYA

When I was on Weight Watchers, I had a book with point values, and the type was so small in the book, I mistook a half of a pizza for being only three points. I ate pizza every day for two weeks. When I couldn't figure out why I was gaining at my weigh-ins, I told my group about the pizza and even showed them in the book where it said it was only three points. It turned out to be three points for one-twelfth of a pizza! —SHANNON

Q: I'm really not into being surrounded by groups of people when I step on the scale. Do I have to weigh in? Isn't there some alternative to this weekly embarrassment?

3FC: We'll give you the bad news first. Yes, you have to weigh in at the meetings. But the good news is that if you're sticking to the plan and losing weight, you're not going to feel embarrassed to step on the scale, you're going to feel proud and excited. It's tough in the beginning, we admit. But you'll be glad to know that it isn't really a public weigh-in, per se. Nobody will see your weight but the weight recorder. The number on the scale is not visible to other members, and it will never be mentioned out loud. In some classes, the scale is even segregated so that nobody even sees you get on it. And you can count on your Weight Watcher leader to be sensitive and compassionate about the process. Your fellow classmates will be too. We've all been there, or are there right now, so you should feel supported, not humiliated, no matter how much you've gained or lost each week.

Many of our Weight Watchers chicks have learned to have a lot of fun with the weigh-ins, and they get a few good laughs with each other to boot, which of course is not only therapeutic but also burns a few calories. You'll be relieved to know that the weigh-ins usually start thirty minutes before the meeting begins, so you can get there early and weigh while nobody is around. If you still really have a problem with the weigh-ins, you might consider joining Weight Watchers Online.

conquering the weigh-in jitters

In the early diet stages, when we are still wearing around the middle a few of the doughnuts left over from our former breakfast life, the thought of stepping on a scale in public is enough to send many chicks scurrying back to the coop. We asked our Weight Watchers chicks to share the rituals that they've developed to help them cope with their weigh-in jitters and climb on that scale every week anyway, to face their personal bottom line, and here are some of their thoughts.

- If they'd let me weigh naked, I would! I can't do that, so besides taking off the obvious shoes, I wear shorts under my pants when it's cold out. I always weigh in with the same shirt and shorts. I take off my pants, shoes and socks, watch, etc. No scarves, retainer, or hair pins, and I don't wear a padded or underwire bra to the meetings!

- I have weigh-in panties. I always wear them to each weigh-in, and I always have a loss. It may sound crazy, but it works!

- I exercise as hard as I can the day before the meeting. The extra sweating helps release any water retention that might be building. Of course no liquids the morning of the weigh-in, so I can get on the scale with an empty bladder! I drink coffee as soon as the weigh-in is over.

- I don't eat my extra weekly points allowance until after the meeting. I generally splurge and use them all at once.

Q: I really like the idea of eating Core, but I don't trust myself to limit myself with eating. If I could do that, I would have never gained weight in the first place.

3FC: Try a combination plan we've come up with called "Flore." Follow the Core plan, but count your daily points. You don't have to do this permanently—just until you feel you can fly on your own. What you do with these daily totals is up to you. Some members just journal in their food so they can see what they *might* have spent on points, had they been on the Flex program. Sometimes just writing down what you eat helps you control your portion.

Other members count their points and stick with their target point range from the Flex program while eating the Core foods, because they don't trust themselves with portion control, but they like the idea of the whole-grain goodness of Core. You can count your intake as you would on the Flex plan, rather than adopting the Core method of trying to set your own limits. We've found that many of our chicks don't feel comfortable with the idea of eating until they're satisfied, because satisfied is a relative term, particularly for those of us in the Captain's Platter Club of life. Sometimes a little external structure and accountability is a comforting thing, so if you don't feel you can do without that structure, don't! But as soon as you feel you're ready to try Core without counting on training wheels, we suggest that you give it a try, since you're going to have to learn how to do this eventually, if you expect to keep the weight off long-term. And why complicate a simple system unless you have to? We do need to mention that our "Flore" plan is not recognized or endorsed by Weight Watchers. This is strictly a member idea.

Q: What is the best way to use my weekly allowance points? I don't want to gain weight. That is a lot of points!

3FC: Don't worry! Be happy! Your target points are carefully calculated to accommodate the thirty-five weekly allowance points, so using them will not interfere with your weight loss. Live it up! Use those points in any way you see fit. Some chicks who feel like they don't get enough daily points even add five points to every day without impeding their progress. They might use them to beef up their breakfast, have an extra snack, or fit in a light dessert each night. Some spend points on a glass of wine and a small serving of dark chocolate, so they can indulge and boost their antioxidants at the same time. Chronic snacker chicks may save those precious five points to satisfy a bad case of the midnight munchies. Others save them up for one special dinner. Some chicks save them for a martini on the weekends, or an elaborate dessert. If staying on plan is hard for you, then you might like to use those extra points as a dangling carrot to keep you on plan for the week. If you know you can have that steak, potato, and dessert on the weekend, you have something to work toward.

To Market, to Market

If you have the munchies but don't have any extra calories to spare, try these one-point snacks and live it up without getting weighed down.

Warning Label: The bang you get for your Flex point buck may vary depending on the brand.

- 1 percent cheese single
- café au lait with ¾ cup skim milk and 1 package sweetener
- 1 cup sugar-free Jell-O and 1 tablespoon fat-free whipped topping
- 1 sheet reduced-fat graham crackers
- 1 cup grapes
- 3 cups low-fat microwave popcorn
- 1 mini bagel
- 1 bottle Yoo-hoo Lite
- 1 fresh peach
- 1 Boca Burger patty
- 2 cups vegetable juice
- 1 cup veggie chips and salsa
- 1 sugar-free Fudgsicle
- 1 Light Laughing Cow cheese wedge
- 1 Eggo waffle

Q: My friend does not recommend that I join WW because she said I can fill up the whole day on low-point junk and not get enough nutrition. She suggests I do something stricter, but I love the idea of the freedom I can have on WW. Any ideas?

3FC: Actually, your friend is wrong. There *are* nutritional guidelines to follow, so you won't lose the day to empty calories unless you break the rules. Points are only part of the program. You need to use the points wisely to get the nutrition you need.

You will have freedom on the plan, but some requirements have been laid out for you, such as the minimum number of servings for vegetables, dairy, healthy fats, and protein. Read your materials carefully so that you get as much guidance from your Weight Watchers program as possible. Even without the guidelines, all chicks should learn to be responsible for meeting their nutritional needs. You may be able to work the system to eat candy bars and spinach salads all day on Weight Watchers, but would you want to?

Q: I am going to eat dinner at my new in-laws' for Christmas and I don't want to make a big deal about my diet. How can I make the most of my feast without blowing it too badly?

3FC: By the time the end of December rolls around, after a month of seemingly endless holiday parties, you are probably ready to throw in the towel and dig in deep. You're smart to plan ahead. This one is tricky! Depending on how your new family cooks, there are various possibilities.

Side dishes are usually not light if they are served as a casserole, so try to take a pass on those if you can come away without looking like too much of a calorie grinch in Whoville. Many casseroles contain cheese, crackers, or creamy sauces, or in our neck of the woods, mini marshmallows. If vegetables are cooked without high-calorie sauces, go for the least starchy vegetable you can find, as the starchier vegetables have more calories.

Hopefully, the entrée is a roasted turkey. You can eat a good-sized portion of skinless breast meat without loading up on calories. The protein will help keep you full longer, and if you're lucky, the tryptophan in the turkey will knock you out until dessert is over. If a salad is being served, get a large portion of it and place slices of the roasted meat on top.

Go light on the bread, and skip the rolls entirely if they're drowning in butter or holiday gravy. Try to add cold salads, but limit portions from ones with mayonnaise in the sauce. Avoid desserts as much as possible. You can clear a day's points in one sweep of the dessert table, so if you do want dessert, limit yourself to one piece or bring one like our Chocolate-Covered Cherry Cake on page 100.

Q: We have a food court at my job, but only one restaurant there has nutritional values listed, and I've eaten there until I'm sick of it. What can I brown-bag that doesn't need to be microwaved?

3FC: If you can carry along an insulated lunch bag, you can generally keep things at a tolerable temperature without a microwave. Try some of these suggestions for a different taste treat that's good on the go.

- Salad with chickpeas, sunflower seeds, light dressing
- Chicken or tuna salads wrapped in a tortilla
- Cold roasted chicken, sans skin
- Pita filled with nonfat cream cheese and berries
- Pasta salad
- Salsa and nonfat dip with raw zucchini or squash
- Grapes dipped in low-fat strawberry yogurt
- Hummus with a sliced pita and fresh veggies
- Bagel with nonfat cream cheese and fruit spread

A thermos with vegetarian chili or light soup or one of our salads on pages 96–98 are also easy to bring along. Pack some whole-grain crackers for crunch. If you're tired of standard lunches, try some snack food like baked chips, light granola bars, or low-fat popcorn.

The moral of this story is don't be afraid to experiment. Break out of your comfort zone, and try some new flavors to tempt your taste buds. Variety will help keep you on plan. Take a risk; it beats eating the same thing every day, and you might find a new favorite food!

Q: I just joined Weight Watchers. I read about a plan on the Internet that will help people break a plateau, and in the plan, you cycle your points up and down every day, with one really high-point day each week. I've written down the formula for my target point range. Is it okay to do it even though I'm not on a plateau? I'd like to try and avoid one, if possible.

3FC: Weight Watchers is one of the most successful diets on the market today, and it is very simple. Give the plan a good try before you tweak it. There has been a lot of research done by professionals to come up with the healthiest and most effective program they can bring you.

Here's a little bit about the theory behind your cycling plan. First of all, cycling has been around almost as long as diets have been around. Many diets rely on cycling to help break a plateau. The goal is to trick the body into releasing fat so it won't think it is starving. By giving it a heftier portion of food unexpectedly, you make your body think the famine is over, and it isn't afraid to burn a few calories. Cycling can be done in many ways, so don't feel you need to follow a specific formula. For instance, you can change your exercise program around. If you've been walking, try doing some kickboxing. Start a weight training routine if you haven't done so already. If you've been doing the same exercise video for months, change it to another one. Simple changes like this will not only break the plateau, but it will make things more interesting for you.

Also, if you utilize your Weight Watchers program as intended, you're probably going to see some cycling regardless. You will be getting activity points for your exercise, which will vary the daily points. You will also get that extra thirty-five weekly point allowance. If you take a special meal or dessert for the bulk of that weekly allowance, you'll practically have your cycling system already done for you.

Q: I've almost hit my goal weight and I don't think I need to go to meetings anymore. What can I do that is more convenient? Should I just get an on-line support group?

3FC: Congratulations on your weight loss! We're betting that the weekly weigh-ins and meetings helped you reach your goal. Our mother taught us to not fix something if it isn't broken. If these meetings have helped you reach your goal, then it makes sense to continue so you can stay at your goal.

Our mother also taught us that weekly meetings are as important to maintenance as they are to weight loss. She goes to her meeting every week, and she's been at goal for three years. She is proud of her weight loss and loves getting free meetings as a reward for sticking with it.

We also know people who have reached their goal through gastric bypass and go to Weight Watchers for weekly support, even though they have to alter the eating plan to make it work for them. They know what millions of other dieters know: Weight Watchers has an outstanding support system, and it keeps them on their toes.

If you continue attending meetings, you will still be weighed consistently and be accountable for your gains and losses. You'll have the incentive of free meetings as long as you maintain your goal weight. You'll serve as an example to others who are trying to reach their goal, and that will be a very rewarding feeling. You'll also share good tips with your co-watchers, learn how to make it through any rough patches you might encounter, and even come home with free, tasty recipes.

Q: I stick to my points, but I'm always hungry! This just can't be enough points for me. I try to spend them wisely. I don't eat "diet cookies" or other junk food that might give me the munchies, so it must mean I need more points. Will I get used to this?

3FC: Congratulations on cutting out the junk food, but you still might be spending your points on the wrong foods. The point values are based on calories, fat, and fiber, but not on food volume. Some foods are denser and have more points for a smaller amount of food. Foods with a lot of water content usually take up more space and are more filling. For example, for two points, you could have a quarter cup of raisins or two whole cups of grapes. Differences like this spawned a diet plan called Volumetrics, which was created by Dr. Barbara Rolls, PhD. Volumetrics teaches us how we can eat lots of high-volume, low-calorie foods and virtually stuff ourselves silly, and all for just a hand-ful of calories or Weight Watchers points. It's easy to apply this logic to any diet plan, including Weight Watchers. Once you learn how to choose higher-volume, lower-calorie foods, you can easily satisfy your appetite and stay within point range.

STRUTTING OUR STUFF

We asked more than a thousand chicks to talk about their best and worst experiences with Weight Watchers, and here's a representative sample of what our chicks are clucking about.

- I can eat chocolate, have a beer, eat Taco John's, etc.; I just have to track my points for the day. I like that it's nonrestric-tive and easy to fit into my lifestyle.
- The flexibility is great. There are *no forbidden foods!* I can eat what I *like*. I have discovered that portion control is not too difficult once you get your mind set right. It has actually opened me up to a wider variety of foods than when I wasn't dieting. My diet consisted of the same basic foods (either massive quantities of unhealthy foods or healthy foods pre-pared in an unhealthy manner). Weight Watchers has actu-ally opened up my world.
- I like getting weighed in. I know that sounds really weird, but if I have a successful week, I'm encouraged by the person who is weighing me. If I don't, they make me feel that I can still keep going.
- The meetings aren't scheduled at convenient times. They don't offer a wide variety of times and days. And they charge you even if you don't attend.

- I don't like constantly thinking about points. I wish I were able to "intuitively" know how much I should eat to maintain my weight . . . and then be able to do so!
- The biggest challenge is to not get bored. I find myself eating the same things because I know the points value.
- I hadn't realized what large portions of food I was eating before. It is hard to keep those under control.

---

weight watchers in an eggshell

Professional Counseling Weight Watchers leaders are not required to be licensed professionals, but they are chosen very carefully. Leaders must be Lifetime Members, and they are hired and trained by the Weight Watchers organization.

Support System Weight Watchers is our favorite support system, bar none. You will be weighed, receive professionally made materials and presentations, and meet other dieters in a nonintimidating, positive, and motivational environment.

Fitness Factor Members are rewarded for exercise by an increase in the amount of food they can eat each day.

Family-Friendly Very! There are no forbidden foods, so you can eat dinner with the family, as long as you exercise portion control. While there is no child care, some meetings don't mind if you bring the little ones along.

* *Continued on next page* *

Pros Weight Watchers has a proven method, with demonstrated success and widespread availability; the plans are simple and easy to follow and emphasize the life skill of moderation, which is essential to long-term success. There is also a Weight Watchers program designed specifically for teenagers. You can read more about these programs at www.3fatchicks.com/weightwatchers.

Cons You can eat a lot of junk food and still stay in your point range. Meetings are only once a week and you have to pay for meetings even if you miss them.

$$ Somewhat expensive. Weekly meetings start at eleven dollars and up. Some locations sell books and accessories, at reasonable prices.

The Person This Diet Is Best For A chick who has other people to please at the dinner table, or a chick who doesn't like too many restrictions or external control.

recipes from the front lines

You can put this strata in the oven to reheat before your morning regimen, and it will be hot and ready to go out the door with you to the meeting. Bring one for a friend, or reheat leftovers another time.

blueberry french bread breakfast pudding

Serves 2

1 large slice (1 ½ ounces) French bread
2 teaspoons cream cheese
2 tablespoons blueberries, fresh or frozen
¼ cup egg substitute
2 tablespoons half-and-half
2 tablespoons skim milk
1 tablespoon maple syrup
Liberal dash cinnamon
Dash nutmeg
Nonstick cooking spray
Additional maple syrup or powdered sugar (optional)

The night before serving: Spray 2 (1 cup) ramekins with cooking spray. Cut bread into ½-inch cubes and divide into two portions. Take one portion and divide it evenly between the two

● *Continued on next page* ●

ramekins. Place one teaspoon of cream cheese on top of bread in each dish. Top with remaining bread cubes and set aside.

Combine remaining ingredients in a small bowl and blend well. Pour mixture over the bread in the ramekins, and slightly press mixture down. Cover each dish tightly with aluminum foil that has been sprayed with nonstick cooking spray. Refrigerate overnight.

The next morning: Preheat oven to 350°F. Bake covered dishes 20 minutes; remove foil and bake an additional 20 minutes, or until golden brown and firm to the touch. If desired, sift powdered sugar over tops, or serve with additional maple syrup.

Per serving: 3 WW points, 144 calories, 4 grams fat, 21 grams carbs, 1 gram fiber, 6 grams protein

If you can brown-bag your lunch, here are a couple of salad recipes that let mayo take a break without giving up flavor. Your taste buds will feel like you cheated, but your thighs won't!

sour cream chicken salad

Serves 2

2 cups romaine lettuce, chopped
2 chicken breasts without skin, cooked and cubed
½ cup roasted red pepper, chopped
6 tablespoons nonfat sour cream
½ teaspoon lemon juice

Salt and fresh ground pepper, to taste

2 tablespoons almond slivers

Place half the lettuce in a small bowl, or into a plastic container, if packing your lunch.

In a medium bowl, add the cubed chicken and red pepper, and toss until mixed. In a small bowl, add nonfat sour cream and lemon juice, and mix thoroughly. Add sour cream mixture to chicken and pepper mixture. Mix gently, to keep from smashing the chicken cubes. Add salt and pepper to taste.

Place half the chicken salad over each of the two servings of lettuce. Top each with half the almond slivers.

Per serving: 5 WW points, 227 calories, 6 grams fat, 10 grams carbs, 2 grams fiber, 33 grams protein

tuna potato salad

Serves 4

7 ounces canned tuna in water, drained

16 ounces canned diced potatoes, drained

¼ cup corn kernels, cooked

2 tablespoons roasted red pepper, chopped

2 tablespoons minced onion

1 teaspoon Dijon mustard

1 tablespoon white wine vinegar

2 tablespoons olive oil

2 tablespoons nonfat chicken broth

In a medium bowl, combine tuna, potatoes, corn, roasted red peppers, and onions. In a small bowl, combine remaining in-

● *Continued on next page* ●

gredients to make dressing. Toss dressing with tuna mixture. Good at room temperature or chilled.

Per serving: 4 WW points, 198 calories, 7 grams fat, 18 grams carbs, 3 grams fiber, 15 grams protein

---

Here's a recipe you can use whether you are on the Core plan or the Flex plan.

salmon cakes with red pepper cream

Serves 4

1 pound salmon fillets
1 teaspoon whole peppercorns
1 wedge lemon
1 medium potato, scrubbed and baked until done
½ cup diced onions
¼ teaspoon salt
Black pepper, to taste
½ teaspoon dried dill
2 egg whites
¼ cup cornmeal
½ cup roasted red pepper
½ cup nonfat sour cream
1-inch piece green onion, white part only

Preheat oven to 425°F. Spray a 9 × 13-inch pan with cooking spray and set aside.

In a large saucepan, bring a few inches of water to a boil. Add peppercorns and lemon wedge and turn down to a simmer; allow to simmer 5 minutes. Add salmon fillets and simmer 10 to 15 minutes, or until done. Remove salmon to a medium mixing bowl and set aside until cool enough to handle. Break salmon into small pieces.

Mash the baked potato in a small bowl. It should yield about one cup. Mix in the onion, salt, pepper, dill, and egg whites. Add mixture to the salmon in other bowl and blend well.

Place cornmeal in a dish. Form salmon mixture into eight patties using about ⅓ cup mixture per patty. Roll in cornmeal, then place in prepared baking pan. Bake for about 20 minutes, then turn patties over. Bake an additional 10 minutes, or until patties are lightly golden brown.

Make Red Pepper Cream:

Combine sour cream, red pepper, green onion, and salt in a food processor or blender. Whirl until well blended.

Serve each patty with a dollop of red pepper cream.

Per serving: 4 WW points, 104 calories, 3 grams fat, 20 grams carbs, 2 grams fiber, 20 grams protein

---

Here's a good recipe that our mother got at her Weight Watchers meeting! Our whole family loves it, even the ones who aren't on a diet.

miss wilma's ambrosia

. . . .

Serves 8

15-ounce can fruit cocktail, packed in light syrup
12-ounce can pineapple tidbits, packed in juice

● *Continued on next page* ●

11-ounce can mandarin oranges, packed in juice

2 small boxes Jell-O brand sugar-free instant pudding mix,
   white chocolate flavor

1 cup fat-free sour cream

6 ounces Cool Whip Lite

Drain the liquids from the cans of fruit and reserve 1½ cups juice. Mix the reserved juice with the pudding mix, using a hand mixer. Beat for 30 seconds. Mix in the sour cream until blended, then fold in Cool Whip. Add fruit and stir to combine well. Chill for a few hours before serving.

Per serving: 3 WW points, 168 calories, 3 grams fat, 28 grams carbs, 1 gram fiber, 3 grams protein

---

Here's a dessert you can bring to any holiday party and no one will know you're counting points!

chocolate-covered cherry cake

Serves 16

16 ounces water pack canned cherries, drained

1 box milk chocolate cake mix

¾ cup Egg Beaters

¼ cup applesauce, unsweetened

¼ cup canola oil

½ cup cocoa powder

1 cup brown sugar

1½ cups boiling water

Preheat oven to 350°F. Spray a 9 × 13-inch baking dish with cooking spray. Spread cherries over bottom of dish; set aside.

Combine cake mix, egg substitute, applesauce, and oil in a mixing bowl and blend with electric mixer until well blended. Pour batter over cherries in pan.

Combine cocoa and brown sugar, blending well. Sprinkle mixture evenly over top of cake batter. Carefully and evenly pour the boiling water over the cake mixture. Place in oven and bake about 30 minutes, or until a cake tester inserted near center comes out clean. Do not insert cake tester all the way to bottom. Remove pan and cool slightly before serving.

Cake will make its own chocolate cherry sauce at the bottom! If desired, serve with a dollop of fat-free Cool Whip.

Per serving: 5 WW points, 227 calories, 6 grams fat, 41 grams carbs, 2 grams fiber, 3 grams protein

Words to Live By

Fat is not a moral problem. It's an oral problem.
—JANE THOMAS NOLAND

My doctor told me to stop having intimate dinners for four unless there are three other people. —ORSON WELLES

5

chicks by the pound
LA weight loss, jenny craig, eDiets

No CHICK IS really an island, but when it's late at night, and the family is sleeping peacefully in the arms of a blissful sugar coma, while we're trying to fight off yet another chocolate and creamy nougat craving, many of us can start to feel like we're stranded on an uncharted desert isle in the middle of the diet ocean. And it's these isolating, Three Musketeers moments that send many of us rowing frantically back to the comfort and companionship of empty calories.

Dieting can be a lonely experience, and sometimes the most important weapon in our weight-loss arsenal is not a pair of running shoes or a bag of carrot sticks or a diet book, but a community of people who are all on that same uncharted isle with us, who can toss us a calorie-free life vest or remind us that we're not alone.

This kind of support is the basis of subscription diet programs like LA Weight Loss, Jenny Craig, or eDiets. These weight-loss plans offer a built-in cheer squad as part of their program, as well as a coach. Subscription programs will hold your hand through every pound. Some programs offer group meetings; others provide one-on-one support. Some diet services even include prepared food. With subscription programs, you can expect to be encouraged, inspired, and guided through every step of your weight-loss journey. They want you to succeed and will usually pull out all the stops to get you to your goal weight. Of course, all of this goodwill and hand-holding will also involve your letting go of some of your hard-earned money.

Why would you want to pay for help and support while you're losing weight? Can't you just follow a healthy menu and get a little exercise and seek out some support for free? Well, yes, you can. And in fact, this is what actually works best for most people. Research has shown that most people who lose weight and keep it off do so by doing their own thing. They don't sit in rooms confessing their darkest dark chocolate secrets. They don't stand on a scale while Nurse Ratched scrutinizes their progress. They don't have their meals delivered every day.

Some chicks, however, who either have busy lifestyles, find zero support at home, or lack the willpower required to beat those late-night chocolate cravings, need the structure, planning, and support that subscription plans provide in order to be successful. And that kind of success is worth more than money.

Weight-loss centers and services are popping up all over the country. Some are good, some are good and expensive, and others just want to lighten your load by lightening your wallet. It's very important, therefore, to do your research before joining a subscription program. Investigate all your options, and read all the fine print in any contract before forking over your cash. We talked to some of our chicks by the pound who have tried some or all of these programs, to find out what they had to say about the good, the bad, and the ugly sides of subscription diet programs.

meet the chicks by the pound

Jennifer from Ohio

I wasn't heavy as a kid, just kind of a bigger girl. When I finished school, I tried several times to get rid of the excess weight, but nothing seemed to work for me. I had limited success with Weight Watchers but didn't learn how to eat properly. I finally got up to 234 pounds and decided enough was enough. I had a friend at work who had amazing success with LA Weight Loss, so I decided to give it a try. I started the program in September, and I lost nearly 40 pounds by Christmas, although I've been a little stalled since then—partially because I exercise too much, and partially because sometimes I cheat. This is a plan and program I feel I can live on for the rest of my life, a true lifestyle change that I haven't been able to make in the past.

Samantha from Ohio

The Jenny Craig program may seem expensive at first, but what you get in return is priceless. Let them take over, and you will lose the weight! Having a personal consultant made all the difference for me. I never succeeded at dieting before, because I needed someone to push me along. I got that with Jenny Craig.

Leslie from Massachusetts

I absolutely love the articles on eDiets, and the best part of this diet program is that you can chat on-line with members from anywhere. At Weight Watchers you have to go to meetings once a week, but with eDiets you can talk to other members anytime you want. I find that solid support has been the biggest factor in my weight loss. In two months I have lost ten pounds safely and without starvation diets or

• *Continued on next page* •

strenuous exercise. It is also more personal and confidential chatting with someone on-line as opposed to going to a meeting where I might feel judged or where I might compare myself to other people.

Marie from California
I like eDiets because it is much more focused than other on-line support resources; it feels more like a community than just a random bunch of people thrown together. I got involved in one of the Challenges they offer and became a team captain. It was my commitment to the team that led to a deeper commitment to the diet/exercise plan and resulted in my losing thirty pounds that I've kept off for a year now.

Marilyn from Colorado
I find eDiets has helped me tremendously to stay focused and obtain my goal. I love not having to go out in rain or snow to be weighed each week, and I can check in on a daily basis versus once a week at a meeting. I have met many interesting people who keep me on track daily. I also love the option to try their various diets and switch plans at any time. If I reach a plateau, I just try switching plans. They also have an excellent support and maintenance board.

LA WEIGHT LOSS

LA Weight Loss Centers are one of the fastest-growing franchises in America. Glitzy advertising campaigns promise an 85 percent success rate and weight losses averaging in the neighborhood of two pounds per week until you reach your goal weight. Who could ask for anything more? But yet, there is more.

LA Weight Loss offers several basic low-fat, calorie-controlled diet plans to choose from, based on your current weight as well as your weight goals. Members receive one-on-one support from a consultant three times a week at their local center. And the plan will work if you can stick to it. Sound too good to be true? Well, here's the fly in the pie. LA Weight Loss is one of the most expensive diet programs available, and it generates more negative feedback than any other diet plan in our henhouse. Here's why.

Expensive program fees and the high-pressure sales of protein bars and other products make this diet hard for a lot of our chicks to swallow. Furthermore, LAWL bases their success rates on "internal audits" not available to the public, so we don't really know what their criteria are. There are no published studies to prove their claims.

LAWL offers six weight-loss plans, called "color plans"—orange, red, blue, purple, yellow, and green—which vary in total daily calories. Food choices are based on an exchange system. You can have a certain number of servings of proteins, vegetables, fruits, dairy, fats, and starches. You are provided with lists of acceptable foods for each food exchange, so you never have to wonder what you can eat—as long as you prepare your own meals. You are also given a list of frozen dinners and selected fast-food items, along with their corresponding exchanges. On the plus side, the LAWL program calls for regular supermarket foods, and includes a detailed manual with a food list that leaves nothing in question. So far, so good, right? Well, just wait. Along with the normal foods, you are also encouraged to purchase LA Lites protein bars and other products, which can really add up. This is where they get you. The bars cost $14 per box of seven bars, and you are supposed to eat two boxes each week.

LA Weight Loss fees average $7 per week. This may sound very affordable, especially since Weight Watchers charges around $13 per week and you don't even get one-on-one counseling. The crucial difference is that you pay Weight Watchers one week at a time, and you choose how long you wish to remain a member. If you don't like the plan, you can leave and find something that suits your lifestyle better.

LAWL takes the opposite approach. You may pay only $7 per week, but you pay the entire amount up front. Your sales rep (aka consultant) will help you determine a goal weight and how many pounds you should lose. They assume you will lose two pounds per week. If you need to lose fifty pounds over twenty-five weeks, you will be charged $175 up front. *Plus* you will also be pressured to purchase a six-week stabilization period and a one-year maintenance period, also for the same $7 per week. Your $7-a-week program now will cost you a nonrefundable $581. But wait, there's more!

Your LA Lites protein bars will run you $1,596, which includes the two boxes per week until maintenance, when you drop to one box per week. You may be offered a discount on the bars if you buy in bulk. Total cost to lose fifty pounds is actually $2,177 plus the cost of groceries.

The average weight loss with Weight Watchers is also two pounds per week. At $13 per week, your total cost to lose fifty pounds would be $325 plus the cost of groceries. Once you reach and maintain your goal weight, you can attend meetings for free as a Lifetime Member.

Has the sticker shock hit yet? Then you're probably coming to your senses and wondering why anyone would choose LA Weight Loss over Weight Watchers. It wouldn't be our first choice, that's for sure. Some of the LA Weight Loss chicks on our forum liked the constant encouragement they received from the thrice-weekly meetings. Some feel that if they pay such a large amount of money in advance, they will be motivated to live up to their commitment. Many chicks really enjoy the one-on-one counseling and learn how to just say no to those pricey protein bars. Other chicks were taken by surprise by the high fees and then couldn't back out or felt so pressured they couldn't say no to the costly frills.

We talked with current and former LAWL members to get the scoop on why they love or hate programs like LA Weight Loss.

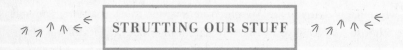

STRUTTING OUR STUFF

The Chicks Sound Off on Subscription Diet Programs

THE BEST THINGS ABOUT SUBSCRIPTION DIET PROGRAMS

• You will always have a support system at your disposal, whether in a group meeting or one-on-one.

- Professional dietitians create the meal plans, so you know you will be eating a balanced diet.
- Support sessions can be a lot of fun and make dieting less stressful and less lonely.
- Some programs include all of your food. Zap it in the microwave, toss the dish in the trash, and you're done. What could be easier?
- You are not pushed out of the nest as soon as you reach goal. Most programs walk you through a maintenance period so you will be prepared to keep the weight off.

WHAT TO WATCH OUT FOR
- Some plans call for long-term, very expensive contracts.
- Additional purchases of foods or products may be required and can be costly. Always check the fine print.
- Don't put too much stock in the white coats. Most counselors are not health professionals but can be former clients or any Jane or Joe who walked in off the street. Make sure you are comfortable with that, and save your health questions for your physician.
- If the plan isn't for you, it may be difficult to get out of your contract or receive a refund.
- You may not like to be weighed by other people.
- Even without a long-term contract, these programs require a regular flow of cash. If you can't afford to keep it up, you may fail the program.
- If you don't like your counselor, you may not be able to switch to a new one.
- Exercise is an important part of any weight-loss program. Some programs never even mention the word. Find out how exercise fits into your new plan before you begin.

Q: I like the counseling and the LAWL plan, but I'm going to have to tap into my kids' college fund to pay for the LA Lites bars! Can I still join this program?

3FC: If you can't afford the bars, or just plain don't want them, then by all means, don't buy them! This is a free-market economy after all, and you don't need the bars to make progress toward your goal weight. There is nothing special in those bars that will speed up your weight loss. We promise. We've talked to quite a few LAWL members who do just fine without the bars. Others choose alternate, less-expensive protein bars that are available in health food stores and supermarkets. Luna Bars seem to be a favorite replacement. They are very similar to LA Lites in nutritional value but cost just a fraction of the price. Another option is to check out eBay, where LAWL expatriates go to unload their surplus supplies. Stand up to the peer pressure, and tell your consultant to mark your file so they don't try to sell products to you again.

To Market, to Market

LA Lites Alternatives

If you don't want to buy the LA Lites but still want to include protein bars in your diet, you can buy less-expensive bars at your nearest health food store or on-line. The general rule of thumb for choosing substitutes is to look for approximately 180 calories, four grams fat, at least eight grams protein, and less than thirty grams carbohydrates. Come as close as you can to these numbers in the substitute bars that you buy, and you will be fine. Our LAWL chicks suggested these as possible alternate bars for you to choose from. Browse your health food store for more options. Most of these bars cost about half the price of LA Lites.

- Luna Bars
- AdvantEdge Morning Energy Bars
- Myoplex Lite Bars
- Powerhouse Nutrition Lean Brownie
- Sugar Free PowerBar Protein Plus
- Optimum Nutrition Complete Protein Diet Bars
- Slim-Fast Low Carb Diet Breakfast Bars

Q: I've started exercising and lifting weights and love the results! I'm losing inches, but the scale is barely budging. My consultant is upset that I'm not meeting my two-pound weekly goal. Should I stop exercising?

3FC: The rules on exercising while on LAWL seem to vary from center to center. Some members tell us they are encouraged to exercise in order to accelerate their weight loss. Others told us they were specifically told not to exercise, because any muscle gain could keep them from meeting their weekly goal. No one should dispute that exercise is good for you. It not only helps tone you during your weight loss and therefore burn more calories, but it helps you to keep the weight off later. Many LAWL chicks tell us that their success is judged by the scale only and not by inches or body fat percentage. We think you should insist that you be allowed to exercise. No one wants to be a flabby chick, no matter what the number on the scale says!

Q: I'm miserable after only four weeks on LAWL, and I want to jump ship. I need a plan that offers more flexibility, which I know I can stick to. What if I can't get out of my contract?

3FC: This is the reason prepaid diet plans are never a good idea. You probably don't know what is going to work best for *you* until you try it. It will probably be very difficult to get out of your contract with LAWL. If you paid with a credit card, you might be able to request a charge-back. Otherwise, you are stuck. You might try the plan again, but allow yourself a few healthy cheats. More than 60 percent of the LAWL members we surveyed said they cheated sometimes and still lost weight. Some people have told us that they couldn't stick with the diet plan and tried a different diet with more success, but continued to keep their appointments with their consultants since they paid for them already and positive support is always helpful. Keep in mind, though, that the consultants are not health professionals but sales reps who are paid commissions based on products they sell to you. If they are not selling anything, they lose some of the motivation to help you. Hopefully, your personal experience and your LAWL support system will be a positive one, and you can combine the consultations with your own diet for your success.

LA weight loss in an eggshell

Professional Counseling Far from it. Your counselors are usually trained in sales, not support, and may have never had to lose a pound.

Support System Regular one-on-one support with your counselor.

Fitness Factor Varies depending on your center. Some push it, some discourage it.

Family-Friendly Yes. The meals are balanced and you can use regular supermarket foods to create family-friendly recipes.

Pros The diet plan is nutritionally balanced, though nothing special.

Cons More focus on high-pressure sales than on support. Reps are encouraged to sell you something every time you walk through the door.

$$ Mind-numbingly expensive.

The Person This Diet Is Best For A chick who needs constant encouragement or pushing to stay on plan, and who has money to burn.

JENNY CRAIG

Just like Joy Behar and Kirstie Alley will tell you, Jenny Craig does it all for you. And she really does. Jenny plans. She cooks. She'll even deliver your meals right to your front door. Jenny tracks your weight, encourages you to stay on plan, and is there 24/7 when you need a little extra support. When it comes to weight loss, many chicks feel that you just can't find a better friend than Jenny.

With the Jenny Craig plan, you can visit your consultant and purchase your food in your local center. If you don't have a center near you, you can use Jenny Direct, which ships your food and offers unlimited counseling by phone. Basically, the only thing Jenny won't do is wash your fork after your meals. In fact, the only difficult part about the Jenny Craig program is paying for it. Food, products, and service plan fees make this program suitable mostly for chicks who have very thick wallets to go with their thick waists.

Food costs average between $80 and $120 per week for the full plan, which includes three meals and three snacks every day. If you have your meals delivered through Jenny Direct, you will also pay a delivery fee. Individual entrées can cost up to $6 each, which is about double the cost of a Lean Cuisine meal at your local supermarket. Satisfaction with food quality seems to vary widely from chick to chick.

Variety also seems to be an issue, as many Jenny chicks get bored after the first month. Jenny Craig introduces an average of three new dishes every year and retires less-popular options at the same time. You will supplement your Jenny meals with fresh fruits, vegetables, and dairy products that you provide. When you are about halfway to your goal weight, you can start providing your own meals one or two days a week, so that you learn how to feed yourself properly. But for the most part, you'll eat strictly Jenny Craig foods.

We have never joined Jenny Craig, but we wondered what "a day in the life of" would be like, so we ordered a trial package. Breakfast was a handful of multigrain cereal, which was tasty but not filling. Thank goodness Jenny recommends supplementing meals with fresh fruit and vegetables. We thought the cheese curl snacks were pretty good; they were lightly seasoned, not greasy, and didn't turn our fingers orange. We also tried a soup and a vegetarian dinner. The potato and garlic soup received mixed reviews. Our Jennifer shuddered and couldn't get past the second bite, believing it tasted too artificial. Suzanne enjoyed hers and thought it was definitely a step up from supermarket soup. The pasta fagioli contained a vegetarian sausage, soybeans, kidney beans, a small amount of pasta, and a specially seasoned tomato sauce. It sounded good, but it also received mixed reviews. Jennifer, transported to her childhood, smiled from fond memories that she couldn't quite place or describe. Suzanne cleared that up for her in three words: Chef Boyardee Beefaroni. Dessert was a small bag of tiny cookies that looked like they came straight out of a Happy Meal. Overall, we thought the food was okay, but it did not convince us to give up our regular diets and convert to Jennyism.

The fees for Jenny Craig are high, and this is a crucial factor for many prospective Jenny chicks. You will pay for a support plan, plus the cost of food. The Gold Plan is the lower-priced option, around $200, and covers support for six months. The Platinum Plan is the more expensive program, about $365, and lasts either a lifetime or three years, depending on the rules in your state. Both plans include one-on-one support from your consultant, either in a center or over the phone. There are no group meetings, à la Weight Watchers. You get personal attention from your consultant, who will offer suggestions and encouragement to help you reach your goals. And Jenny frequently offers short trial memberships at a low cost, so you can try them out before you commit to anything long-term.

For the most part, the Jenny Craig program is well planned and leaves little room for error. They literally do everything for you, from meal planning and cooking to cheering you along. This plan is appealing for anyone who needs strict structure or convenience. Most people probably won't need this level of hand-holding. Those who do need it and can afford the program usually stick it out long enough to see some significant weight loss.

The number one complaint we've noticed is the expense of the food. Most Jenny Craig members are very happy with the program, though there are a few out there who have less than positive experiences to share.

Q: I just started the Jenny Craig program but am not sure I can afford the meals. Lean Cuisine dinners cost about half of what Jenny meals cost. Can I buy my own food and still be successful?

3FC: Part of the success of the Jenny Craig program stems from the fact that they control your food for you, until you learn how to make better food choices on your own. Plus, because Jenny provides in advance only as many meals and snacks as you'll need, you don't have an unlimited supply and are not likely to overeat. Besides, at these prices, who can afford seconds? Being on Jenny Craig is a little like being stranded on an island: you know the next airdrop of food will not come for two more weeks, so you make your supply last. If you know you can hop on a raft and go to the next island for more supplies, you may be more inclined to eat additional foods that you don't need. The high price you pay is not just for the food but also for the external portion control and the peace of mind that comes from letting somebody else make the hard decisions for you.

When you are halfway through the program, you can move to Halfway Days, where you buy only part of your food from Jenny, the rest from your local supermarket. By then you will have learned enough about self-control to be in charge. You will also be motivated by the weight you've lost to stay on track, but until then it's a good idea to stick with Jenny.

If your budget or your appetite truly can't wait, try buying a small quantity of frozen dinners to keep on hand, and see how you do. Your Jenny Craig counselor understands budget issues and will work with you. You will also need to be aware of the exchange system and make sure the new meals fit in your program. Your counselor will help you to gradually increase the frequency of your own meals until you feel comfortable that you are in charge and are not going to hop on a raft and row in the direction of the nearest all-you-can-eat luau.

Q: I joined Jenny Craig to lose weight for my class reunion, and I worked hard to reach my goal. I ignored the advice of my consultant and ate strictly Jenny Craig food the entire time to make sure I met my goal quickly. It paid off when all of my classmates were surprised by how hot I looked! Now that the reunion has passed, I've tried to keep the weight off, but I can't seem to make the right choices. I'm quickly regaining the weight. Will I have to re-join Jenny for life just to keep the weight off?

3FC: The Jenny Craig program makes it easy to lose weight, because they do everything for you. At some point, though, you have to learn how to take control of your eating, and this is where the Halfway Days come in. Jenny teaches you how to eat, but you have to do your part too. You skipped a crucial phase in your weight-loss journey, which would have prepared you for maintenance. Talk to your counselor about going back, and don't take any shortcuts this time.

Consider rethinking your goals, as well. Reunions, weddings, and other special dates are fine for smaller short-term goals, but they don't keep you motivated after that magical date has passed. Think about how much healthier you feel now. Make it your goal to keep that feeling long-term. Above all else, don't let go of the wonderful feeling that you had at your reunion. You were a hot chick then, and you can stay that way!

Q: I love the packaged entrées and soups, but my whole family hates vegetables and we never eat them. Even President George H. W. Bush refused to eat broccoli! My counselor says I need to change my habits and eat more veggies because the entrées alone are not enough.

3FC: It may not have been the broccoli that moved President Bush to ban it from White House menus and even Air Force One; it might have been his broccoli chef. Bland, overcooked veggies are certainly not a meal for a president, or a fat chick on a diet! But if you experiment with cooking techniques and seasonings, you may be surprised with what you come up with. Many of our members have shared tips for improving on Mother Nature when it comes to vegetables. We *love* oven-roasted vegetables and veggies cooked on the grill. These methods bring out new, richer flavors that you didn't know were there. Condiments such as soy sauce or some of the Jenny Craig sauces are also perfect for adding new depth to the flavors in everything from broccoli to zucchini. Don't be afraid to experiment!

Q: I'm bored with the food selections in Jenny's kitchen. It's becoming more and more difficult to stick to the program. What should I do?

3FC: Boredom can be a real diet buster! There are several things you can do to add variety to your meals without straying from plan. It's better for you to keep eating the Jenny Craig foods, but you can change them somewhat by seasoning with spices or Jenny-approved sauces. Make use of the list of unlimited free foods; for instance, add some roasted red peppers to the JC chili, to add sweetness and additional flavor. Consider using a Jenny Craig cookbook to prepare, with your consultant's advice, recipes that will fit into your plan. Freeze leftovers to liven up another boring day. If you think more creatively in the kitchen and the market, you will eat more creatively.

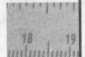

jenny craig recipe for success

Since Jenny cooks all of your meals for you, you'll never have to don an apron in the kitchen. So instead of offering a recipe for this diet plan, we thought we'd share a few ingredients to help make this plan a success!

• If the meals become monotonous after a while, try changing your environment instead. Buy a few special dishes, a new tablecloth, and even pull out the candles and music. Make your meals seem like special treats, even if this is the seventh time you've had Jenny's Personal Pizza this month!

• Take advantage of your counselor—in a good way. Never skip a session, use all the time you have available, and don't be afraid to open up about your diet concerns or slipups. Your counselor's goal is to help you succeed, so let her.

• While Jenny doesn't offer an exercise plan, you can try an on-line program like www.eFitness.com, join a gym, or just get out and stroll the neighborhood. The important thing is to get moving and not just depend on the diet to get you to goal.

• Birds of a feather flock together. Look locally or on-line for other Jenny Craig members and make new diet buddies. You can share insider tips and advice that you won't find anywhere else.

Q: I'm apprehensive about joining a plan where I will have to see a personal counselor, but I also think I need someone to seriously kick me in my 4X pants. This is embarrassing. I don't even want anyone to know how much I weigh. Will I have to share my weight and eating habits with a lot of people?

3FC: Don't worry; you won't have to weigh in with a group of people on Jenny Craig, just your consultant. You can also ask to see the same consultant every time if it makes you more comfortable. Don't think twice about letting them know how much you weigh. They can probably make a good guess just by looking at you, anyway. Many JC consultants are former clients, so chances are that they were once a 4X too! The first weigh-in is always the hardest. You'll come to look forward to future weigh-ins because it's an opportunity to see the pounds drop off. Don't be afraid to jump in there. Take off your shoes, jacket, jewelry, and spit out your gum, then hop on that scale! Get to know your consultant and make her your best friend away from home. Blurt it all out, honey, and make the most of it, because you're paying for it, and Jenny's one-on-one support doesn't come cheap. Try to overcome your fears and take full advantage, so you are sure to get your money's worth.

jenny in an eggshell

Professional Counseling Sort of. You can see your counselor any time or have access to a counselor 24/7 by phone. However, they are not health professionals; they are usually people just like you who have lost weight and know the Jenny Craig system inside and out.

Support System Just the one-on-one support from your counselor. You can join their free on-line forum if you want support from other members. You can find more Jenny Craig resources at www.3fatchicks.com/jennycraig.

Fitness Factor Exercise is encouraged, but they do not offer a specific exercise plan. You're on your own.

• *Continued on next page* •

Family-Friendly No. All meals come in little single-serving packages. You'll still have to cook for the rest of your family.

Pros Meals are prepackaged, so you can't overeat. You never have to worry about what you should or can eat.

Cons You don't learn how to make your own choices until you are halfway to goal, when you are allowed to have occasional meals on your own. Meanwhile, what will you do if your FedEx shipment of food gets diverted to Alaska? Additionally, the food isn't all so fabulous.

$$ Very expensive. The food costs make Jenny Craig one of the most expensive diet plans available.

The Person This Diet Is Best For The chick who doesn't like or need to cook, doesn't want to worry about planning meals, and doesn't mind paying for the luxury.

---

eDIETS

The eDiets plan is an interactive on-line dieting program that you can mold to fit your lifestyle. It is totally Internet-based, which is handy for many of us who are shy about stepping on a scale in front of a crowd each week. The eDiets system has a well-rounded approach to healthy weight loss, including menu plans, recipes, support groups, and fitness plans. Their Web site can be overwhelming at first thanks to the massive amount of content available; however, if you give it a little time, you'll be finding your way around quickly. This program simplifies much of your diet, whether you initially choose a program that works for you or you need to switch diets. If you want to eat vegetarian, low-carb, or low-fat, or even just delete a certain species from your diet, you can let eDiets do the work for you. You can choose from eDiets' own programs, or you can choose a commercial plan that they have incorporated into their program, such as Atkins, Eating for Life, or Bob Greene's Total Body Makeover. We've been waiting patiently for eDiets to include a Krispy Kreme or a Burger King plan, but that hasn't happened yet.

The great part about eDiets is that you can change your diet plan anytime, as often as you want. It's a very flexible approach to dieting. If you check out a menu and see that it isn't for you, just click to another diet plan to find a menu you can live with.

The core of eDiets is the total nutrition planning that they create for the dieter. The dieter inputs her weight, goal weight, height, activity level, and a few more pertinent items, and then chooses from one of the many diets that are suggested. Based on your weight-loss goals, a plan will be developed for you with the proper amount of calories. Then eDiets creates your entire menu and even a shopping list for the next week, based on your individual practical and physical requirements, including satisfaction and convenience. You can even choose meals from fast-food restaurants for any meal of the week. Sounds easy, but what if you don't like what they plan for you? Just click a button and you can choose from a list of substitutes. Just print your shopping list and you're all set!

Like all good diet plans, eDiets recommends regular exercise. Their fitness section will help you plan a workout regimen based on your goals and abilities. It also shows you how to do exercises with a virtual trainer. And take it from us, he's really inspirational. We accidentally left our screen on, and when we came back three hours later, he was still doing sit-ups. Just imagine the virtual abs he must have! If you don't like or cannot do one of the prescribed exercises, you can trade it for another one. Just like the eMenus, the exercise routines offer great flexibility.

On eDiets you can also get a full-course support system. If you subscribe to this section, you will have access to message boards for all of the plans they offer, plus special boards created for group efforts, motivation, exercise, recipes, and more. Chat rooms are also available, and eDiets has chats scheduled several times a day so you can chat with the eDiets staff and guest speakers on various subjects.

Finally, there is an exhaustive recipe area on eDiets. If you subscribe, you will have access to over 2,000 diet-approved recipes. Here you can print recipes and compile grocery lists for your chosen dishes. This is a big time saver, so you can more easily fit in all those exercise sessions you've been putting off!

The eDiets program is going to cost you anywhere from approximately two to ten dollars a week, depending on how many extras you choose. We've all been spoiled at some point by freebies on the Internet, but sometimes you really do get what you pay for.

Q: I just signed up to eDiets, but there is no way I can afford to eat like this. The cost of produce and all of the extra meat is just too high for my budget.

3FC: If lean meat, fruit, and vegetables seem too expensive, then perhaps you need to take a closer look at your household budget. If you've been feeding your family boxed dinners and family-sized budget frozen dinners, then yes, maybe you will wind up spending a little more for fresh, quality food, but consider what you'll be eliminating from your budget each week. No longer will you have to dip into your wallet for indulgences like chips, ice cream, cakes, burgers, pizza, soft drinks, candy, alcoholic beverages, or frozen snack foods. And because healthier food means healthier bodies, you will probably spend less in medical costs. Besides, health is always a sound investment and can mean the difference between paying the grocery store now or the cardiologist later. And cardiologists cost a lot more than broccoli.

how to eDiet without going eBroke

Here's a few tips from our eChicks about how to stay on plan, and on budget.

1. Pick one snack from your menu and repeat that through the week. It's cheaper to buy one or two items to split for several days than to buy five cartons and barely touch them.
2. Buy your vegetables at a farmers' market or roadside stand. Save money and get fresher ingredients.
3. Purchase frozen produce when possible. Stock up during sales and cut your produce expenses in half compared to fresh produce.
4. Choose recipes that use beans and tofu for a meat replacement. You can save up to 75 percent of your entrée expenses by doing this.
5. Buy the Sunday paper each week to check the sale pages. Find the one grocery store that has the best overall savings based on your grocery list.
6. After you print your shopping list, go through your cabinets and see what you already have, then mark that off your list.
7. Buy spices in bulk at a co-op or your local health food store. A small scoop in a baggie can be bought for mere cents, compared to several dollars for a full jar.
8. Buy large quantities of freezable foods when on sale. To keep organized, date each item with a freezer marker before placing in the freezer, and mark it again when you thaw it.
9. Don't buy specialty products. Bars, shakes, candy, or "diet" brands can often be replaced by similar products.
10. Experiment with substitutions. If raspberries are four dollars a pint, try two-dollar strawberries instead.

Q: I can use free message boards all over the Internet. Why should I pay extra here to chat at eDiets?

3FC: You are right, there are many large, free message boards on the Internet, including 3fatchicks.com! Personally, we three chicks are as happy as pigs in mud at 3FC, however, with eDiets you will have the convenience of having this message board at your fingertips while you are checking your menu, entering your statistics, or choosing a workout routine. You may be more inclined to visit them, and participate in them, if you are a paying customer. We've always found at 3FC that more involvement with our support group helps us stick with our program in the hard times.

Unlike many free support systems, eDiets has several chats each day with professionals from various fields, like registered dietitians, psychologists, and fitness trainers. We've found that these chat rooms are not utilized nearly as much as they could be. In many circumstances, the chat rooms are nearly empty, and sometimes chats are even canceled for lack of attendance. These are prime opportunities to pick the brains of the minds that can help you succeed. The eDiets site has a paid staff, so you are paying for their licensure and knowledge. Free sites, such as ours at 3fatchicks.com, have volunteer administrators and moderators, who are less likely to cut your meat for you before you eat it.

Q: I find eDiets always has something for sale, and the last time I bought something, I got a lot more than I bargained for. This was kind of a turnoff. Are they really interested in helping me drop my pounds or just my money?

3FC: Certainly eDiets can seem a lot like a virtual shopping mall, and there are plenty of ways to click away your hard-earned cash. This is, after all, an extensive site with many licensed professionals on staff to pay for. Weight loss is a billion-dollar industry, and people who are in this business are in it to make a profit. But that doesn't necessarily mean that they aren't offering a valuable service, and of course, moderation isn't a bad idea when it comes to shopping either.

The program's one-stop shopping design, which allows you to do all your diet-related business in one place, is part of what makes eDiets so popular. The eDiet "mall" includes not only support and planning, but a store offering diet foods, snacks, exercise equipment, videos, books, supplements, and beauty products. This is ultraconvenient for busy chicks who just don't have the time to shop around and don't mind paying a little more for the convenience.

And, of course, dieters are prone to impulse shopping for diet products, so we make great customers. Just be cautious and, as you're learning to do during a Big Mac attack, try to control your impulses. There may be fifty ways to lose your blubber, but you only need to try them one at a time. Just because you signed up for a new diet doesn't mean you need to buy multiple diet foods, exercise videos, magazines, supplements, and cookbooks. Take it one step at a time and don't burn up your resolve—or your budget—in the first two weeks.

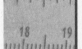

buyer beware

Seventy-one percent of chicks who left eDiets did not think it was worth the fee or were unhappy with other financial practices; however, when we sampled eDiets ourselves, we found it to be rather straightforward regarding costs, and we had no surprises when the credit card bill came. With any on-line purchase, though, you need to read what you are buying. The most common complaints among our eChicks:

● The initial fee is $1.99 a week, but subscribers did not read that it was billed quarterly and were unpleasantly surprised to find $25 on the credit card statement.
● Dieters signed up for the main plan only, but when checking out, found the premium plans in the shopping cart. These plans had to be deselected or would be purchased. Some di-

● *Continued on next page* ●

eters clicked through without paying attention and unintentionally bought the larger packages.

- Some dieters were not happy that all of the programs were billed separately. The plans looked inexpensive, but they added up when purchased.
- Some felt that they were tempted with diet candy or similar products while searching the site for support to get past their sweet tooth and snacking issues.
- Dieters felt that it was too easy to buy the extra products because their billing information was stored in their account; in a weak moment they could make impulse purchases without ever leaving their chair.

Q: Why shouldn't I just print my menus or buy frozen dinners and quit? I can do the same thing on my own.

3FC: One of the things that we eChicks love most about eDiets is the convenience of having meals that are readily available and easily changed. You can make changes right up to mealtime. You can even change the whole diet plan right up to mealtime. Having such a flexible program, which will conform to fluctuating moods, helps you cater to the finicky chick in us all and makes it less likely that we will quit. In our view, that is worth every penny we spent. After you have been on eDiets for a few weeks, you just might get the hang of it and be ready to start doing things on your own. If you do, just be aware that you've lost a solid support system, accountability with weigh-ins, the assurance that your daily calories are balanced and nutritious, along with all of the multiple resources that were at your fingertips on eDiets. Make sure you can find replacements for these as well, or you may find you aren't as successful with your weight loss as you had hoped.

eDiets recipe for success

We tried to come up with a smashing meal for eDiets, but the only recipe we could find that was acceptable on all plans was boiling water. Instead, here are our best tips for using eDiets to help you succeed at weight loss:

1. Utilize the meal plans for restricted diets. Sometimes when we don't have a lot to choose from, meal planning can look bleak, even though we have many possibilities before us. For instance, when Suzanne tried Atkins, even though she had a fridge full of acceptable foods, she could only manage to come up with salad for breakfast one morning. If she had had eDiets, she might have had mock French toast or a basil frittata!

2. Maximize your fitness possibilities through on-line chats with eDiets' own personal trainers. Are you stuck in an exercise rut? Don't know the difference between a Swiss ball and a medicine ball? You can get a fresh new approach to fitness and find answers to any question you may have in one of eDiets' scheduled chats.

3. Do you need a helping hand to keep you on your diet? Sign up for a mentor. You'll have somebody to help you through the rough patches and cheer you along the way. After you are on the road to success, sign up to pay it forward and mentor someone who was once in your shoes.

Q: When it comes to helping me make good choices at fast-food joints, eDiets is really great, but what can I order when I'm going out to a fancier place?

3FC: You're right, eDiets does a great job helping you to work fast-food restaurants into your meal plan, but they don't list many full-service restaurants, so here are a few pointers from our eChicks, to help you dine out without bombing out.

1. Arm yourself with a restaurant nutrition guide to make your best choices for the plan you are on. Most chain restaurants offer nutritional information if you ask.

2. Go all the way and eat at an elegant restaurant. It will be harder to overeat with ornate stemware and fancy dishes.

3. Keep a couple of small pieces of chocolate by the plate. When you feel satisfied, push your plate back and eat the chocolate. This gets the taste for dinner out of your mouth, and the dessert signals the body that it is through eating.

4. Want seconds? Make it a dinner salad with light dressing, and hold the cheese.

5. Score your plate into halves. When you've finished your half, pop a strong mint or cinnamon gum into your mouth and kill those pesky taste buds for a few minutes. When it comes to eating moderately, Altoids can be your best friend.

6. Find the best-looking waiter in the place, then ask to sit in his station. Stud muffins have zero calories.

7. Ask for vegetables on the side instead of potatoes or pasta. Unless it is a casserole, you are almost guaranteed fewer calories.

8. Ask if the baked potatoes are oiled or buttered before they are baked, and avoid them if they're swimming in fat.

9. Remember that condiments are an accent, not an entrée!

10. Ask your server to bring half your meal on the plate and pack the other half to go.

eDiets in an eggshell

Professional Counseling With your paid subscription, you will have access to dietitians, personal trainers, psychologists, and more.

Support System The program has an excellent chat network and message forum, for an additional fee. You can read more about what eDiets has to offer at www.3fatchicks.com/ediets.

Fitness Factor Motivation and instruction are available to get your body moving, as well as an interactive fitness system that will teach you to exercise.

Family-Friendly Yes. You can pick and choose your menu, plus switch out meal plans for other dishes your family can eat.

Pros A wide variety of diets to choose from. Great daily menus with instant shopping lists.

Cons Everything has a price tag. Advertisements for their extra services at every corner.

$$ It is reasonably priced for the basic program, but all of the options are extra, which can be expensive in the end.

The Person This Diet Is Best For The impatient dieter who hops around to different diets, or the person who spends a lot of time at the computer.

recipes from the front lines

The LA Weight Loss plan calls for a lot of simple but healthy foods, such as lots of vegetables and lean meats, but it can get boring. Here's something to spice up your life—or at least your dinner!

hot and spicy buzzard

Serves 2

½ cup low-carb ketchup (we like Heinz)
¼ cup Worcestershire sauce
¼ teaspoon crushed garlic
4 teaspoons finely minced sweet onion
¼ teaspoon dry mustard powder
1 teaspoon dried thyme
¼ teaspoon coarse fresh cracked black pepper
1 extra-large buzzard breast (may substitute 1 pound boneless, skinless chicken breasts if buzzard is not available)

Preheat oven to 350°F. Combine all ingredients, except buzzard, in a small bowl. Place buzzard in a glass baking dish and rub half of sauce over the breast, turning to coat, and reserve remaining sauce. Cover dish with foil and bake for 20 minutes. Remove foil, turn buzzard over, and continue to bake for an additional 20 to 30 minutes or until breast tests done. Spoon remaining sauce over breast and serve. Be careful, it bites!

Words to Live By

I haven't trusted polls since I read that 62 percent of women had affairs during their lunch hour. I've never met a woman in my life who would give up lunch for sex. —ERMA BOMBECK

A positive attitude may not solve all your problems, but it will annoy enough people to make it worth the effort. —HERM ALBRIGHT

fit chicks

8 minutes in the morning, body for life, curves

EVER SINCE JANE FONDA encouraged us in her *Complete Workout* series to "feel the burn," some of us chicks have been pulling out the spandex and the leg warmers and the color-coordinated sweatbands to start programs that emphasize exercise, rather than diet, as the main focus of our weight-loss strategy.

Most other diet plans focus on the food and build in enough activity to make sure you don't eat more than you can burn. Exercise-driven weight-loss programs, however, take exercise to a new level; they help you lose weight through targeted and regular activity, accompanied by diet guidelines.

When you actually put down the remote control and go to select an exercise-driven diet plan, though, things can get kind of confusing. When you first enter the world of commercial fitness, you can feel like you've just landed on Planet Infomercial, full of enthusiastic bumper stickers that promise everything from radically improved health to instant beauty to spiritual enlightenment in no time flat. "Work out for just thirty minutes, three times a week, and realize your wildest weight-loss goals!" "Transform your body, your mind, your spirit, inside and out, in just twelve easy weeks!" All these glowing promises can really make a fat chick's head spin. So how do you determine who is telling the truth and who is trying to sell you some prime swamp land in Florida?

We've found that when it comes to the glowing adjectives and purple promises of the weight-loss industry, it's best to take a step back and look at "just the facts, ma'am." And fact number one is that regardless of the weight-loss plan you choose, you are going to have to exercise. Yes, it's true; you have to move to lose. And we've heard all the excuses, so don't even bother. We know it's difficult to work all day, cook, clean, take care of kids, shop, run errands, and do all the other things that life calls for. However, the fundamental laws of physics say that if we don't exercise, we aren't going to live as long, as happily, or as healthfully as we could.

We three were never too crazy about exercise. And that is an understatement. Until just a few years ago, our experience with exercise was limited to two items. One was a pink spring-loaded contraption we squeezed while we chanted, "We must, we must, we must increase our bust!" The other was a stylish brown nylon rope thingy connected with pulleys that hung on our doorknob. We attached all of our limbs at once, and "toned" ourselves by pulling them back and forth. We mostly just got our heart rate up by screaming, "Don't open the door!" whenever anyone walked by.

This must sound like the typical "When we were your age, we had to walk ten miles to school barefoot!" And, in fact, that's not far off, because we really are living in a new and improved fitness world. These days, fortunately, there are plenty of programs and devices that are exciting, convenient, efficient, and effective, and you won't wind up on the wrong side of a door jamb.

For one thing, gyms aren't the high-pressure scenes that they used to be. There have also been a lot of improvements in gym culture, which is good news for all of us timid gym bunnies who have been shying away from fitness centers because we remember the high-pressure social clubs of the eighties. There is still some socializing, and some pretty staggering six-pack abs, but overall, people in gyms are answering a health alert these days, and not a booty call.

There are also women-only facilities now, and hospitals now feature wellness centers frequented by doctors and other health-related employees, who are there, by and large, for the health benefits. What safer place to test your limits on a treadmill than surrounded by cardiologists! And of course, there are great programs you can do right in the privacy of your own home.

Whether you are selecting an exercise-driven weight-loss program or just an exercise program that will complement your diet-driven program, here are some things we think are important to consider:

- Pick a program that emphasizes fat burning, not just weight loss.
- It's best to find a regimen that is designed or at least has been tweaked for a woman.
- Some programs offer options or solutions for larger women with special fitness needs.
- If you're just starting out on a fitness regimen, pick a program that's good for beginners but offers room to grow.
- It's important to find a plan that emphasizes balanced nutrition for overall fitness and energy levels.
- Always consult with your doctor before beginning any fitness regimen.

And bear in mind . . .
- Results are not always quick.
- Fitness requires dedication and perseverance. If you slack off too soon, you will lose any benefits you gained and end up at square one again.
- Be patient. You may have to experiment to find the right combination of diet and exercise to be effective for you.

- Some plans, like Curves, may not grow with you as you lose weight and increase your fitness level, so you may need to change programs or join a traditional gym.
- Since you will be building muscle as you burn fat, you may not see a dramatic drop in pounds, but you will lose inches. If you want to see progress, instead of stepping on a scale, check yourself with a tape measure or watch your clothing sizes drop.
- Reaching your goal weight doesn't mean that you're finished. Maintaining a fit body with exercise is a lifelong commitment. Use it or lose it.

In this chapter, we will guide you through some of the most popular weight-loss fitness programs available today: 8 Minutes in the Morning, Body for Life, Body for Life for Women, and Curves. To help us get our finger on the pulse of these popular programs, we asked our fit chicks to share some of their thoughts and experiences about what worked and what didn't work for them.

Although there are positives and negatives to all exercise-driven weight-loss programs, one thing is true no matter which regimen you choose: when it comes to exercise, there are no excuses! Some studies show that around 90 percent of women who lose weight and keep it off long-term do so by incorporating exercise into their diet programs. Those who stop dieting and exercising after they reach goal often regain their weight. Exercise isn't a temporary solution, it is a commitment, and the benefits are countless! So the good news is that much of the hype you hear and read is true. You really can protect your bones, fight your flab, boost your metabolism, burn calories, help ward off disease, improve your sex life, and find greater peace of mind, all through regular exercise. And all you have to do is get up off that couch and start moving to the music!

meet the fit chicks

Ilene from Ontario

At forty-eight, I am in better shape than I was in my late twenties, when I first discovered exercising after quitting smoking. Presently I run and weight-train three to four times a week. In the summer I bike and Rollerblade too. Exercise, along with eating five to six healthy meals per day, has kept my weight stable. I love to see people starting an exercise plan and I am especially happy when I see that they enjoy it and are eventually hooked! I'm an exercise junkie now and I want everyone else to be one too. Make sure the exercise you do is fun though, because it is for a lifetime!

Tiki from Michigan

I've had success in the past doing just cardio, but I ended up with a smaller, squishier version of me and that isn't what I want. I want nice leg muscles that can help me teach my cheer team their jumps, strong arms so I can do push-ups with my son, and the exercise that builds my muscles will also help to build my bones and protect them from osteoporosis. With strength training, I'm down from the 170s to 156. The goal is a solid 135. I like having some curves on my body.

Jo from Wyoming

I was overweight simply because I got too busy doing other things and failed to pay attention to what I ate. I am finding maintenance difficult since old habits die hard. It is nice to be a smaller size, to be able to do more things, and to be able to shop in the ladies department rather than the XXX sizes. And above all things, I do not want to regain any of the weight I have lost. I joined Curves for Women and am enjoying it. This past year I went through a series of radiation treatments. I am convinced that eating properly and exercising regularly helped me through it all. I formed the habit of going directly to Curves for my exer-

• Continued on next page •

cise right after each radiation treatment. That was a good stress buster. At seventy-nine years of age, I believe that we can lose weight and maintain that loss at any age, and we can keep smiling along the way.

Melanie from Pennsylvania

I'd heard of a program called Body for Life, which was based on heavy lifting and eating six small meals a day. The before-after pictures promised me exactly what I wanted. We had plenty of weights at home, so I started. A few weeks into Body for Life, I realized I was probably going to maim myself doing this at home without proper gym equipment. I found a fantastic trainer, now my boss, who at fifty-seven years old is a true testament to the fact that the fountain of youth is found in a gym. He taught me how to eat, how to work out, how to design my workouts for specific goals, and how to just keep on doing it, day after day, year after year. After four months of my new program, my weight was still 135, but I'd dropped from a size 8/10 to a size 6. My body fat dropped from 27 to 22 percent. My trainer suggested I get my certification and come work for him. Me? The ex–fat lady? I've been working as a personal trainer now for two years and love it. I wear a size 2 to 4, my body fat is 15 to 16 percent, and I've maintained my weight at 125 pounds.

↗ ↗ ⋀ ⋀ ⇐   STRUTTING OUR STUFF   ↗ ↗ ⋀ ⋀ ⇐

Melanie Gumerman is a certified personal trainer. She is also a part of the 3FC team and moderates our fitness forums. We asked Melanie what we could gain from hiring a personal trainer.

Melanie

I love seeing my clients succeed. I train women, men, older adults, weight-loss clients, athletes, rehab clients, fibromyalgia patients. Picking goals and milestones is crucial to success and to long-term success-

ful maintenance. If I didn't keep setting goals and doing something I enjoy, I wouldn't still be doing this. I've learned through the years that a trainer can help in so many more ways than the obvious ones. Here are just a few of the benefits you gain from working with a personal trainer:

- Education about the proper technique and form for an exercise so that you don't get hurt and you do work the muscles that you think you are working.
- A program that is specifically designed to meet your individual goals.
- An understanding of how to put together your own workouts with alternate exercises if you don't want to or can't afford to always work with a trainer.
- The ability to set realistic long-term goals and plan how to get there.
- Accountability and a reason to show up at the gym.
- Ongoing support and new exercises and training modalities as your fitness level or interest changes during your fitness journey.

We have learned that personal trainers are not only more affordable than we thought but often crucial to keeping their clients on an exercise program. A short-term contract with a trainer, or even occasional sessions, could mean the difference in success or stalling. An experienced trainer can accelerate your weight loss!

JORGE CRUISE: 8 MINUTES IN THE MORNING AND THE 3-HOUR DIET

For all of us busy chicks who don't exercise because we don't have time, the Jorge Cruise program claims we don't have to put off the inevitable any longer. Because after all, who doesn't have just eight minutes in the morning to devote to better health?

Okay, we know this sounds a little far-fetched, and in fact, we were a little skeptical ourselves and probably never would have even tried this plan if Mr. Cruise hadn't been such a hottie. As it turns out, Mr. Cruise's theory does make sense and does work, although once you read between the lines, you will see that there is more to the program than those golden eight minutes in the morning.

This plan works best for newly hatched fit chicks who don't exercise at all. It's a palatable program that helps start fitness beginners on the road to better health. On this program, you will start each day with a quick, energizing "Cruise Move," tone your muscles, and boost your metabolism to burn more calories all day long. What isn't emphasized in the title, however, is the considerably longer time you'll spend power walking three times a week to maximize your weight loss.

Mr. Cruise's diet plan is not very well delineated. We are given general guidelines and a few basic nutritional dos and don'ts. After that, you're left to fend for yourself. Most of the 8 Minute chicks we surveyed thought the plan wasn't specific enough with regard to diet. Cruise has since solved that problem with the addition of another book, *The 3-Hour Diet,* which encourages you to eat healthy foods every three hours.

The book *8 Minutes in the Morning* isn't intimidating, as other fitness books can be. The photographs inside are not of skinny, superfit chicks. Cruise promotes not getting skinny but getting healthy and feeling better, which are more positive and realistic goals.

Unlike many other diet and exercise programs, Cruise helps us to deal with the emotional aspects of dieting and weight loss as well. You are encouraged to love yourself and cultivate a positive self-image. Cruise considers self-esteem to be the key to the success of his program, and we agree that every dieter should pay more attention to the self-love aspects of the weight-loss process, because when you feel better about yourself, you just automatically start to look better.

The core of 8 Minutes in the Morning is the exercise program called "Cruise Moves." Cruise Moves are designed to help firm your muscles as well as boost your metabolism when you're at rest. According to Cruise, lean muscle mass is what controls your metabolism. Your body burns between 20 and 50 calories for each pound of muscle, every day. So, his theory goes, if you increase your lean muscle mass, you burn more calories. If the Cruise Moves firm up five pounds of lean muscle within the first few weeks, you could burn an extra 250 calories per day. This equals more than twenty-five pounds of fat loss per year. This is a good tip, no matter what diet and exercise plan you follow! During this phase of the daily program, you will exercise for eight minutes every morning. Each day you will focus on a different body part, so that your whole body has had a good workout by the end of the week. Eight minutes of exercise is definitely doable, but if you are using the Cruise plan as your weight-loss program, don't start whistling "Dixie" yet. Cruise also suggests thirty minutes of power walking three times a week, to exercise your heart and burn even more calories. Realistically, we all need sixty minutes of exercise a day to maintain and ninety minutes a day to lose, but many people can't commit to that kind of time without any previous exercise experience.

The 8 Minutes in the Morning program seems to work great for our fitness newbies because it's quick and easy and not intimidating. And let's face it, eight minutes of exercise a day is better than nothing, and hopefully it will give newbies a positive taste for exercise and push them to do more. Some of our more seasoned chicks felt that this program didn't hold up too well for them over the long haul and felt that they needed more exercise after the first few months. A whopping 34 percent of the chicks we surveyed didn't lose any weight at all on this plan and left for another program, such as Weight Watchers or Curves.

So to get the real skinny on the 8 Minutes in the Morning program, we asked our fit chicks to air in on their experiences with the charismatic Mr. Cruise.

Q: My first month doing 8 Minutes was great. I actually lost weight! Months two and three were not so good. I'm still cruising but not getting anywhere. I do my eight minutes every morning; I follow the Cruise Down Plate and just eat the foods in the book. Is this program just for beginners?

3FC: Yes and no. Many of our members felt that this program was best for starting out, and they later moved on to join gyms or other fitness programs that pushed them more. That's not a bad thing. Getting in shape is a positive lifestyle change, no matter which way you slice it. And just as sitting on the couch only leads to lying down on the couch, exercising generally leads to the desire to do more exercise. So try to do a little more and see if it boosts your weight loss. Maybe you aren't exercising as much as you could be right now. You didn't mention power walking, and Cruise suggests a good half hour three times a week. This may be the boost your body needs to start burning more weight.

Another suggestion would be to look more closely at your food intake. If you follow the guidelines in the book, you should be right on track. However, eyeballing portion sizes isn't for everyone. A "fistful" of anything is a relative term. For one thing, whose fist are we talking about, Shania Twain's or Shaquille O'Neal's? It can't hurt to add up your calories every day to make sure you are eating enough, but not too much. Fit Day is a great Web site where you can track your diet and exercise. Go to www.fitday.com and sign up for a free account for logging your food, and take a few minutes each day to use it. You might be surprised!

To Market, to Market

Best Food and Fitness Trackers

If you feel that keeping track of calories every day is about as much fun for you as math class, you might consider nutrition software that tracks your daily intake. These newfangled programs can make dieting fun and easy, and you're sure to make a perfect score every day. Many even let you enter your activities so you know how many calories you burn. Most offer free trial periods, so you can try before you buy.

- FitDay, www.fitday.com. Choose between a basic, free on-line version and a deluxe software program to purchase and install on your own computer.
- Diet Power, www.dietpower.com.
- ProTrack, www.dakotafit.com.
- Balance Log, www.healthetech.com.
- Check out www.3fatchicks.com/onlinetools for reviews of the newest diet and fitness software.

Q: I'm having trouble with the portion control approach in the Cruise Down Plate program. I know how to count calories. How do you know how much is too much?

3FC: Cruise suggests that we practice portion control, because it's a natural way to control consumption. Once you learn how much is too much and how little is too little for your body, eating moderately becomes a lot easier than counting every calorie every day for the rest of your life. But it can be a little difficult getting a handle on this new approach at first. Here's how it finally boiled down for us. Take a standard nine-inch dinner plate and mentally divide it in half. Fill the upper half with vegetables. Then mentally split the lower half into two sections. Fill one of those with meat or other high-protein food, and the other with carbohydrate foods. Cruise offers suggestions for each food group. Add a fat, preferably flaxseed oil, which helps your body to function and also helps curb your appetite. Now, clean your plate! If you are still hungry, eat more vegetables. It's not as easy as it sounds, though. There *are* foods that need to be measured, but you can quickly learn to eyeball those amounts too. Cruise recommends eating three meals and two snacks per day, which is typical of most balanced diet plans. He also recommends finishing each day with a delicious dessert. You'll always be full, and you'll never feel deprived.

If you need something more structured, Cruise's new book, *The 3-Hour Diet,* fills the bill. Unlike his *8 Minute* series, this book focuses on diet rather than exercise. This time we are told to eat every three hours, and we can have snacks such as candy bars and potato chips and have fast food for dinner. You are encouraged to eat *something* every three hours, to keep the metabolism revved and burn more calories, even if that something is one sugar-free cookie or fifteen fat-free potato chips. However, this is still very much a diet. Recommendations include small portions, fat-free cheese, and sugar-free gelatin. Fast foods include grilled chicken, plain burgers, and salads with lemon juice or nonfat dressings.

Q: I understand the fitness part of the 8 Minutes program, but there isn't enough info on the diet. I'm so confused about what to eat! Can I just follow another diet plan, like Weight Watchers, and do the fitness part according to the book?

3FC: Absolutely! It is recommended that you follow the diet guidelines in the book, but it's not required. Of course, if your vegetable for the day is a piece of sweet potato pie swimming in brown sugar and marshmallows, you're not going to lose weight. But if you're reasonable about your diet, you will see the benefits of exercise as long as you are consistent with the fitness portion of the program. Don't stress yourself out over the diet plan in the book. If you haven't looked at *The 3-Hour Diet,* you may find it easier to follow than the guidelines in the *8 Minute* books. The important thing is to find a diet that you are comfortable with, so you'll stick with it.

Q: The 3-Hour Diet includes a treat such as candy every day so we don't feel deprived. My problem is that I don't trust myself to have it in the house because I'll eat it. I could make a bag of cookies disappear in only eight minutes!

3FC: You aren't alone. It's difficult to keep candy and other treats in the house, considering that overeating and even a little lack of control is what got most of us fat to begin with. If the book recommends one quarter of a bag of M&Ms, how easy is it to resist eating the rest of the bag? First of all, it's okay to choose a snack that isn't so tempting to overeat, such as yogurt, fruit, or veggies. If you want a cookie or one Reese's Cup, we suggest you store the rest in the freezer. If you do sneak into the bag, you might change your mind before the extra portion thaws out. Better yet, don't even buy it in bulk packages. Take the time to drive or walk to a local convenience store and buy just one single-serving-sized snack. The extra trip may be annoying at first, but it will pay off in the end.

snack on this!

The 3-Hour Diet and 8 Minutes in the Morning allow two snacks a day that could be sweet or salty treats that you probably thought you had to give up entirely. If you don't trust yourself not to overeat, try these snack ideas that offer easy portion control.

- Browse the snack aisle for kid-sized snack packs. You'll find treats, such as gummi-bears, in small packages designed for packing in lunch boxes.
- Bake your own brownies using a low-fat brownie mix or one of the delicious recipes from www.3fatchicks.com. As soon as they are cool, cut into small squares, wrap tightly in plastic, and put them in the back of the freezer.
- Don't be put off by the extra cost of individually wrapped portions. They're usually cheaper than a binge.
- Go ahead and buy a full-sized candy bar from a vending machine at work. Score points with a coworker by cutting it in half and sharing.

Q: My 8 Minute Moves are the perfect thing to get me started each morning, but I fizzle out pretty quickly. I work in an office all day and don't have time to eat. I'm tired and hungry when I get home, and just the thought of a power walk leaves me exhausted. Am I destined for the slow lane?

3FC: It doesn't matter what diet plan you are following, you need to eat during the day. You can't cruise on empty! All of Jorge's books recommend three meals and at least two snacks for a reason. It may not be convenient to eat an apple or go out for a salad, but there are a lot of quick and easy foods that will sustain you until you get home. Snack on nuts, Pria bars, or other fast snacks suggested in the books. Lunch doesn't have to be time-consuming, as long as you prepare it before you even leave the house. Pack a cooler with everything you need to quickly assemble a sandwich or salad at your desk. It's easier than you think. Within a few days, you'll find that you have so much energy, you may even want to power walk all the way home! Pita sandwiches make the perfect lunch on the go. One pita half has just seventy calories! Stuff with a garden salad, peanut butter and jelly, fruit and cream cheese, or even scrambled eggs and bacon. Pack any wet fillings in a small plastic container, and fill your pita at lunchtime.

8 minutes in an eggshell

Professional Counseling Limited. You can subscribe to the on-line service and pay for premium support. You won't get one-on-one counseling, but you may get to join a live chat with Jorge himself!

Support System Paid subscription to on-line service includes community support forums where you can get encouragement and advice.

Fitness Factor Absolutely! You'll exercise every day and learn the importance of fitness in the weight-loss equation.

Family-Friendly Not really. Most of the meal ideas are designed for one person. Fitness is also often a solo experience.

Pros Doesn't require much time, plus everything about exercise is spelled out for you. The diet is vague, however, which was a problem for some chicks.

Cons You may outgrow the exercise routine quickly, though that isn't exactly a con in the big picture!

$$ Cheap! Other than the cost of the book and maybe a pair of dumbbells, you don't need any special equipment. Suggested meals are very affordable. If you opt for the on-line service or premium support, though, the cost can quickly add up.

The Person This Diet Is Best For The fitness newbie, the single person, or anyone with very little time to devote to fitness.

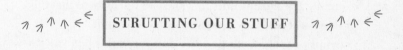

STRUTTING OUR STUFF

The Heavy Hens Air In on Fitness

Let's face it: exercising while obese is not easy! You may not be able to do the same exercises as thinner women. You may have problems bending over and getting up quickly, and your

• *Continued on next page* •

joints may hurt from the extra weight. You may have difficulty using some kinds of exercise equipment. You may also feel self-conscious exercising around other people. But it can be done, and you really will be glad later. We've been there, and we will share our best tips, and those of the heavy hens in our community, to help you get started.

- Check with your doctor before starting. If you are obese, you have a higher risk of heart disease or high blood pressure, so you may need to be monitored during an exercise program.
- Don't worry about starting slow. You can graduate to more traditional exercises as you gain strength and lose weight.
- If you can't walk for a full half hour, try ten-minute walks, three times a day.
- If weight-bearing exercises, such as walking, are too hard on your joints, try swimming or water workouts. If you feel too self-conscious for the pool, check your local wellness center. Some offer water classes just for overweight women.
- Do push-ups against a wall or the back of a chair.
- If chafing from exercise is a problem, try one of the new body lubricants, such as Body Glide or Soothing Care Chafing Relief by Monistat, to prevent friction.
- Leakage may be a problem, because of the extra padding pressing down on the bladder when you do sit-ups or other exercises. Use a panty liner for now, and rest assured that this problem will probably go away as you lose weight.
- If sit-ups put too much pressure on your back when you do them on the floor, try doing crunches while lying on a balance ball.
- When choosing fitness equipment, be sure to ask about the weight limit, especially on budget-priced models. Many treadmills and elliptical machines were not designed to hold more than 250 pounds. There are a lot of better-quality machines that will hold you now and will provide many years of

fitness. You might even try a Gazelle or other glider. These machines are very low-impact and great for getting started.

BODY FOR LIFE

Body for Life (BFL) is a body-sculpting and weight-loss program that is adaptable to almost anybody. The program is led by Bill Phillips, a formerly overweight man who is now sporting a dramatically healthy and chiseled body. BFL, which recently had a makeover, now has a version exclusively for chicks, called Body for Life for Women, led by our new hero, Dr. Pamela Peeke, who understands that fitness really can be feminine.

Body for Life, promising "12 Weeks to Mental and Physical Strength," encompasses positive thinking, a balanced eating plan, and a cardio and weight training program. Keep reading! Don't let the weights turn you off. BFL is one of the most intensive "weight lifting for weight loss" plans, and it will build muscle, but having muscle tone doesn't mean you're going to be bulky. Trust us. Fat rolls feel a lot bulkier than strong muscles do.

The point of the Body for Life plan is to lose fat, not muscle. According to Bill, half of the weight lost in a typical diet is muscle tissue. By lifting weights, you save and develop muscle tone, which means you lose more pure fat.

The Body for Life program is broken down into a few major components. First we learn how to Cross the Abyss. Don't be worried if you're afraid of heights. This abyss is a psychological one, and it represents our need for a mental transformation to change our mind-set if we are to achieve our goals. This section of the book is probably not the most popular one with impatient chicks, but stick with it, because it will greatly increase your chances of achieving your goal and making it stick.

Here in the abyss, you will identify what your goals are, what you need to do to get there, and what bad habits you have that are likely to hold you back. Talk about a reality check! You'll have to be totally honest with yourself, before you can safely reach the other side.

Be sure you pick goals that are attainable. Climbing to the top of Mount Kilimanjaro before you touch your next Twinkie is perhaps a bit of a stretch, but making a commitment to exercise a little more every day and cutting down on your Twinkies whenever you can is perhaps a little more attainable. Achievable goals are important because you'll be spending a lot of time writing them down, reading them back, and saying them over and over to yourself every night for the next twelve weeks. You don't want to spend the next three months thinking about how you're falling short.

BFL has a wham-bam-thank-you-ma'am approach to exercise. The plan includes twenty minutes of intense cardio three times a week, alternating with three days of forty-five-minute weight-training sessions. That's it. This leaves time for more important things in life, like a little afternoon delight under the spreading magnolias.

We love the Eating for Life section. Here's why: you get to eat six times a day. That's right, six times a day! What's the catch? These are small, low-fat meals, and you have to keep them balanced with carbs and protein. Most meals can be made by measuring a fist-sized portion of carbs and a palm-sized portion of protein, prepared in a low-fat manner. There is no calorie counting. Many of the meals are quick fixes, and the book lists many examples of acceptable foods. You'll choose a protein and a carb for each meal, and you'll add a vegetable to two of the meals. Your meals can be as simple as cottage cheese and an apple or a meal replacement shake. You can also cook regular meals with lean meats, healthy grains, and vegetables. You'll do this for six days, and then once a week you get a free day when you can eat anything you like.

Yes, you read that correctly! We three chicks live in the land of milk and honey-glazed ribs, so we like the idea of being free to indulge in the richness of our culinary heritage without having to pack our bags and go on a guilt trip afterward. You can eat anything you like on free days, but remember, you need a calorie deficit to lose weight, so don't go overboard. Choose foods you can't eat during the week and limit yourself to one serving. Don't go hog wild. Eat just one Moon Pie. Have a half cup of fried okra, not the whole pan full.

We'd be a lot happier if there was a video to accompany this book to show the fluid movement of the weight-lifting moves for those of us who are new to strength training. We also think the program could be improved with a scorching butt routine and more emphasis on food portions, but to get the real skinny on Body for Life, we went to the fit chicks on this program, and here's what they have to say:

Q: I've been on this for four weeks and haven't lost weight. What is wrong? Am I building muscle?

3FC: Although you are building muscle, you aren't seeing results on the scale at this point. It is possible that your muscles are retaining water since they are new at training. This is perfectly normal and healthy. If you aren't losing weight, measure your success in other ways. Are you getting stronger? Were you once topping off with five-pound weights, but find yourself lifting eight- or ten-pound weights now? You should also take your measurements, and take an updated photo of yourself to compare with your starting photo. The scale isn't the only tool to measure perfection. A snapshot can show more results than the numbers between our big toes. When it comes to before and after, a picture really is worth a thousand calories!

If your pictures or measurements aren't very impressive, take another look at your portion sizes. Do you have too many yolks in your omelet? How thick is your palm-sized protein portion? Are you mixing your protein shakes with milk or water? Are your meals more than 20 percent fat? Is your free day sucking up all of the good work you've done the rest of the week? Keep tabs on every bite you eat, and count your calories. Make sure you are eating six balanced meals, spaced apart as directed in the BFL book. Make necessary adjustments and by week eight you should see a big difference.

You might also consider adding extra cardio to the plan to burn more calories. Some of our fit chicks do feel that they don't get enough cardio on this plan, and they incorporate extra cardio sessions throughout the week. We suggest that if you add cardio, don't add more of the high-intensity sessions as outlined in BFL. Instead, add less intensive, but longer, fat-scorching sessions.

↗ ↗ ↑ ⋀ ⇐ | STRUTTING OUR STUFF | ↗ ↗ ↑ ⋀ ⇐

Our Chicks Air In on Portion Control

Does your hand grow when it is time to measure your fist-sized portion of pasta? While some BFL chicks use measuring cups just to be safe, there are some more creative options. Here are a few tips from our chicks to prevent portion overload.

Try baked spaghetti squash in place of pasta. It's awesome and you can eat a ton of it for very few calories! — MEG

Slice or shred cabbage very fine (like you would for coleslaw) and sauté it in a bit of olive oil or pan spray. You can have heaps of it with tomato sauce and browned ground turkey breast or lowfat ground beef, with a sprinkle of Romano or Parmesan cheese. It tastes wonderful and you get a helping that fills your plate and stomach. You can mix in a half cup of whole-wheat pasta if you really want the pasta, but I don't miss it at all. — MEL

I add cannellini beans or black beans and canned artichokes (in water) to pasta to make a full bowl for an "American" pasta meal. I get the taste of the pasta and some extra fiber. I find that a quarter cup of pasta, a quarter cup of beans, three artichokes, plus sauce, is a good meal for me! — ELLEN

Q: I feel like all I eat is oatmeal, apples, and eggs. When my free day comes, I go wild and enjoy myself, but I spend the next few days battling cravings. Is there a happy medium?

3FC: Don't take Free Day too literally. It might be guilt-free because free days are permitted on the diet, but you'll still pay for it in the end. This is your day to eat what you want, but excess calories *will* affect your bottom line. Period. No ifs, ands, or bigger butts. So, if you're about to tuck into some southern-fried comfort food, think twice. Don't go overboard and find yourself with a sugar hangover that lasts for days and makes your diet days that much harder.

As for eating oatmeal, apples, and eggs all the time, you can remedy that by buying Bill Phillips's book *Eating for Life.* There are many great recipes in the book, as well as ideas and tips to help you come up with your own meals. You know you can have a palm-sized portion of meat and a fist-sized carb, so all you need to do is add the spices and condiments and you can come up with a multitude of combinations. One great recipe to try is our Shrimp with Asparagus and Couscous on page 175. If you can conjure up your creativity, then you won't have to rely on Free Day to get you through the week. You can eat satisfying meals all week long and still lose weight.

As you progress through the Body for Life program, your body will become more accustomed to this healthier way of eating, and most fit chicks actually prefer good nutrition and eventually forget Free Day altogether.

> ## *tips for avoiding*
> ## *a calorie blowout*
> ## *on free day*

If you're focusing on Free Day all week long, you're liable to snort cocoa when the big day finally comes. Your first Free Day is the most exciting. You're going to eat whatever you want because, by golly, you've *earned* it. By the end of the day, the sugar coma you've fallen into will help kill the chocolate-induced endorphins—until, of course, next week's Free Day!

Free Day is a wonderful concept, but you don't want one day to untie all of the hard work you've done all week. Remember that calories count! Here are some tips from our fit chicks to help you keep your Free Day fantasies under control.

- Limit Free Day to only one meal instead of a whole day.
- Make a list of what you crave the most through the week. Choose only from that list when Free Day comes around so those foods won't haunt you for another week.
- Don't eat for the sake of it. If what you really want is the french fries, don't buy the burger.
- Eat what you want, but journal every bite and count the calories at the end of the day.
- Don't eat seconds at any meals.
- Weigh in the morning of Free Day.
- Eat six small meals as usual, but eat in any combination you choose. Double up your carbs or add some fat.
- Don't buy bags of Free Day supplies. You don't want them teasing you from the cabinet for the next six days.
- Wear tight-waisted pants while you eat.

- Still drink plenty of water on Free Day, and have a tall, cold glass before each meal or snack.

Q: I'm just not physically strong enough to do this. It's a waste of time, and I can't imagine that I'll ever be able to get results. I even had a hard time getting the dumbbells into the shopping cart.

3FC: Not all chicks were born with golden biceps, but that doesn't mean that trying to work the program is a waste of time! Be more patient with yourself, and work your way in gradually. Start with a set of weights as light as you need. You don't have to start out with fifteen-, ten-, or even five-pound weights. If you need ones and threes, that is a start! It really is okay: you want to challenge yourself but not hurt yourself. You need to build with each set to hit your max on the intensity scale. That will require focus and honesty. Your max will float from one day to the next, especially when you're just beginning. If you can't hit the same weight you did the session before, that's okay. Some days you'll be stronger than others; just keep your focus, and be sure to log in your activity on the journals included in the book.

Jumping from a five-pound weight to an eight-pound weight or from a fifteen-pound weight to a twenty-pound weight can be difficult, particularly across an entire set. If advancing to the next weight seems too hard, buy some single-pound magnetic plates for metal dumbbells from a sporting goods store. Instead of jumping several pounds at once, you can increase one pound at a time and keep steadily advancing.

ladies who lift

I added yoga to my plan, and I now feel like I get a better range with my weights. I was never a flexible person, but yoga has allowed me to get in touch with my body and realize how far I can take it. — PAULINE

When I first started going to the gym, I didn't ask the other people for advice. They are impressive and look good because they concentrate on the weights and don't small-talk much. The talkers are the gym bunnies, and you don't want to be one, no matter how cute the name is. If they see you're serious, they'll offer help where needed. — DANIELLE

I can't get the most out of my workout unless I get plenty of sleep. If I sleep less than seven hours the night before I lift weights, I can't reach my potential. — SANDY

I keep motivational pictures on the wall where I lift weights. I get them from muscle-chick magazines. If I'm having a tough time lifting, all it takes is a glance at the muscles on the wall to keep me going. I also have pictures on the inside of the door to the snack cabinet, which has proven to be very handy! — MARYANNE

Q: I just don't believe it. There's no way I'm going to lose weight with three twenty-minute cardio sessions a week. It's just too incredible to be true. Isn't it?

3FC: Okay, we can understand how you might have misgivings about the extraordinary claims this program makes, but we're here to tell you, this program is *not* too good to be true. The twenty-minute Aerobic Solution is high-intensity interval training (HIIT). It's only twenty minutes, but it is one hellfire session. We three chicks prefer what we call "sorta high-intensity interval training" (SHIIT), but that isn't on this program.

You can tweak the cardio if you feel it will work for you, but if you are not experienced, be careful. Bill has done his homework and has a proven program. If you overtrain, you can actually impede your weight-loss efforts. The general consensus is to not add to the number of intense cardio sessions. Instead, try adding longer, less intense workouts, either in separate sessions or as add-ons to the HIIT sessions. With such a small amount of required cardio, you have plenty of time to explore more activities, such as swimming, belly dancing, kickboxing, or power yoga.

body for life bites

Here's a sample day in the life of a fit chick on Body for Life:

Meal 1 • Oatmeal and scrambled eggs and whites
Meal 2 • Myoplex shake
Meal 3 • Cottage cheese and strawberries
Meal 4 • Turkey and Swiss wrap with fresh green beans
Meal 5 • Grilled marinated chicken breast, baked potato, and steamed asparagus
Meal 6 • Myoplex shake

body for life in an eggshell

Professional Counseling None.

Support System Nothing formal. There are various support groups on the Internet, including the forum at 3FC. Check out www.bodyforlife.com for good tips in the guestbook.

Fitness Factor Exercise is intense but time-efficient. Cardio twenty minutes, three times a week, and strength training for forty-five minutes, three times a week.

Family-Friendly Not very. Most of the meals can be eaten by any member of the family, but you'll be eating smaller amounts of food six days a week. This can be difficult when you're cooking normal-sized meals for a family.

Pros You don't have to cook much on this plan. Super simple to follow.

Cons Video to show form in exercises would be helpful. We've heard many requests to increase cardio in the program.

$$ If you drink ready-to-drink shakes and take supplements, at least your wallet is going to lose weight. Otherwise, the food is cheap.

The Person This Diet Is Best For A single chick or anyone who brown-bags her lunch. Also great for the person who wants to get in shape and doesn't know how.

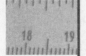

alternachick tips for getting fit

Are you looking for a nontraditional form of exercise to wake up your senses and explore your alternative side? Try these tips from our alternachicks, for new and enlightening ways to get in shape.

- Belly dance. If exotic, sensual dance is more your style than hip-hop aerobics, you might try belly dancing as great way to burn calories and get in shape. Follow a video or join a class to shimmy into shape.
- Dance Dance Revolution. Attach a special dance pad to your video game console, hang a disco ball from your ceiling, then follow along for the most fun fitness workout since *American Bandstand*!
- Yourself Fitness. Computerized personal trainer via PlayStation or your PC. Work out your inner alternageek!
- Martial Arts. From kung fu to Tae Bo, the martial arts offer head-to-toe fitness and extreme calorie burning. *Kee-yah!*
- Yoga. Connect with your body on a deeper level, and intensify your inner motivation while you get more flexible. Try power yoga for more calorie burning and better circulation.

●

BODY FOR LIFE FOR WOMEN

This chickcentric version of BFL takes everything we learned in Body for Life but zeros in on the uniquely female weight-loss experience, which sounded just fine by us! Dr. Pam Peeke, who is obviously a woman, understands that we chicks can get to feeling overwhelmed with the amount of responsibility in our lives. And what chaos doesn't take care of, hormones will. The plan is somewhere between Jane Fonda and hard-core weight training. It's a great mix for any woman, and later on, if you're interested in more weight training or less hard lifting, you can decide which direction you'd like to take. We think this is one of the most sensible and well-rounded diets available.

The book goes through the four hormonal "milestones" of life with us. The doctor's ingenious mantra of "Mind, Mouth, and Muscle" helps us tackle the obstacles we all face during each hormonal milestone.

"Mind" is all about managing stress, taking care of a busy life, and making time for ourselves. It includes ten Power Mind Principles, which will help motivate you, empower you, and build your confidence.

"Mouth" is your new way of eating. The book goes over how to eat, what to eat, and when to eat it, yet the diet makes so much sense, it feels totally unrestrictive. It's very simple. You'll eat three meals and two snacks a day, and the book includes a list of acceptable foods. At meals you will have a portion from the protein list and a portion from the carb list. At least twice daily you'll add in a nonstarchy vegetable, and you are free to add more. You'll use good fats, in low-fat proportions. For snacks, a list of options and portion sizes are available to you.

"Muscle" is the physical portion of the plan. The plan recommends thirty minutes of cardio, at least three to five times per week. You are encouraged to give it your all and to rotate activities. You will also do resistance training three times a week, and the workout is a simple program to follow. You can do the entire program at home, using as little equipment as a few sets of dumbbells. You can round off the cardio and weights with Pilates and yoga.

The driving principle behind this plan is to build up your muscle so you can burn more calories in future workouts. Muscle burns more calories than fat, and if you increase your muscle mass, you will shed more weight by merely existing. How great is that?

One of the best parts about starting Body for Life for Women is that all of these components don't have to be changed at once. Dr. Peeke says that if you want to concentrate on one part at a time, then that is fine with her, although to be successful on this plan, you really do have to get around to reading the whole book at some point. Reading the food and exercise appendix off the Internet isn't going to make this a successful plan. Doing the whole program, you will eventually get mind, mouth, and muscle all working together in perfect harmony!

Q: Is this diet low-glycemic? I am so over low-carb/good-carb. The only thing I lost on those diets was money.

3FC: This is not a low-glycemic diet, but there are "smart carbs" that you will be allowed to eat. You may not have lost weight before because you didn't practice portion control. We love juicy steaks and whole-grain bread, and we are all for any diet that allows these delicious foods, but we also remember that we can't lose weight if we eat a two-pound sirloin and a whole fresh loaf of pumpernickel.

With this plan, you will have a list of smart carbs to choose from. These are carbs that have more nutrients and fiber than their high-glycemic counterparts, such as the whole-wheat pasta in our Seafood Stuffed Peppers recipe on page 176. Brown rice, sweet potatoes, and whole-grain bread are chosen for their nutritional value. As you eat balanced meals with reasonable portions, your goal is to get more bang for your buck with smart choices in foods.

Unlike most popular diet plans on the market, Body for Life for Women encourages you to count calories if you are not losing weight, or if you have a difficult time with weight loss. Serving sizes are given on your food list, so much of the guesswork is eliminated and you don't have to count calories to be successful.

Q: Do I get Free Day on BFL for Women? That was the most enticing part of BFL. The exercise chart says Free Day, but I don't see it anywhere else.

3FC: Yes and no. You will have an exercise Free Day, but as for a total day off from your eating plan, no. Instead of full free days, you are allowed what are called "mini-chills," small nibbles of off-plan foods that you can take to keep yourself in sync without feeling guilty about it.

Peeke says that although you may indulge in many mini-chills at the start of the program, you will probably find yourself going for much longer periods without them later on. There is not a specified amount that you can have, but be aware that whatever calories go in must come out. If you want to lose weight, reserve your mini-chills for those times when if you don't have a cookie or a scoop of ice cream, you are going to begin peeling the wallpaper off the walls. Satisfy yourself with a small portion of forbidden food, and then move on with the plan guilt-free.

tips for boosting your get-up-and-go

We only get one day free of exercise per week. What can we do for motivation those other six days? Here are our top five motivators to keep us exercising when we really want to hit the snooze button:

1. Pencil yourself in. If you schedule your time to exercise, you've made it an important part of your day and you are more likely to stick with it, or at least work harder to think of an excuse.
2. Leave your workout clothes on the dresser. We keep a complete set of exercise gear ready and waiting at bedside so we don't have to search before dawn.
3. Keep a small album of your goal pictures in your gym bag or over the alarm clock. Tack inspirational pictures around the exercise equipment.

4. Announce your victories! Try marking a bright red *V* on your wall calendar on days you stick with the program.

5. Mix it up! Tired of spinning? Try African dance, kickboxing, salsa, or circuit training. Keep it interesting, and keep your muscles guessing.

Q: I've never lifted weights before and I imagine I can't lift very much. I also don't want to look "ripped." Is this program too advanced for me? I looked into BFL before and I didn't think I could keep up.

3FC: This program is made for you! Body for Life for Women is very user-friendly and easily modified for the beginner. One nice thing about the plan is that Dr. Peeke recommends starting with just one element of the program at a time, until you feel you are ready to move on and add the next element.

Muscle, the weight-lifting portion of this program, is as intense or low-impact as you want it to be. So if you're dumbbell-challenged, there is still hope for you. One-, three-, and five-pound weights are okay to start with. You can even repeat one-, three-, and five-pound weights if you want. As long as you are doing all you can do, and truly advancing the weights as you are able, you will still see progress.

And don't worry about looking ripped. A lot of hard work is involved in achieving a body that will make people confuse you with Arnold Schwarzenegger, which is the physique most people think of when they hear "ripped." You will attain a healthy look while on BFL for Women. Just keep going until you get the body you want, and then maintain a holding pattern. The beautiful part is it's all up to you!

body for life for women in an eggshell

Support System Nothing formal. There are various support groups on the Internet, including the forum at 3FC. Check out www.drpeeke.com for additional information.

Fitness Factor Time-efficient and easily modified. Exercise is an important portion of the plan. Cardio is recommended three to five times a week, weights three times a week.

Family-Friendly Fairly easy to do with a family. Meals are smaller than what the rest of the family may eat. You'll have three meals and two snacks a day.

Pros Plan is simple to follow. It's clearly explained in the book, without vague areas. It can all be performed at home.

Cons There are still off-limit foods, like white potatoes and white rice. No videos to follow along with for the novice.

$$ The food can be bought as cheaply as any other plan. Meat choices may be more expensive, but cheaper items, such as cottage cheese, eggs, and oatmeal can make up the difference.

The Person This Diet Is Best For The woman who would like to get into a solid exercise program or who has had problems sticking to a diet. The Mind portion of this plan overcomes a multitude of obstacles and focuses on positive thinking. This is particularly good for women whose weight loss progress tends to be sluggish.

CURVES

Twenty years ago, gyms were as much about socializing as they were about fitness. The gym bunny trend has scared away many a chick who would like to work out but is afraid of being the chunky chick in the middle of a Victoria's Secret or Abercrombie and Fitch ad. Although the gyms of this century are different, chicks across America are finding comfort and safety in Curves, a women's-only workout facility.

We understand that no matter how relaxed today's gyms are, some women just feel intimidated by a gym. We surveyed our chicks and found that the most popular reason for choosing Curves, hands down, was its nonintimidating, all-female environment.

Curves offers clients a diet program as well as an exercise regimen. You are not, however, obligated to follow both elements of the Curves program. You can do either or both at any local Curves facility, or you can buy the book *Curves: Permanent Results Without Permanent Dieting* and do the program right at home.

Curves Diet Plans

Curves offers two types of diets—the Carbohydrate Sensitive Plan and the Calorie Sensitive Plan. Both diets are low-carb; one involves counting calories. You'll take a test to see which diet you need to follow.

The Carbohydrate Sensitive Plan looks eerily like one other low-carb plan that we know of that begins with a scarlet A. This diet starts out with a beginner's phase, where you will get to eat twenty carbs (minus fiber) a day. After Phase 1, you'll move to Phase 2 and raise your carbs to forty to sixty per day. You'll stay at this level until you reach your goal.

The Calorie Sensitive Plan allows for a few more carbs up front, but it adds calorie counting to the mix. In Phase 1, you can have twelve hundred calories and sixty grams of carbs per day. After Phase 1, you'll move to Phase 2 and raise your calories to sixteen hundred per day. The carbs stay at sixty grams. Your calories will not increase or decrease based on your weight.

The Curves diet has a "free foods" list valid for both plans. The list includes one protein shake a day, plus a choice of other "foods." At first glance the list looks long, but it does include garnishes and foods you won't eat much of, like parsley, garlic, mustard, and bean sprouts. Still, it's nice to know there is an arsenal of foods that you can eat that won't be tallied against your daily limits.

Either diet plan should get you to your weight loss goal, which is called Phase 3. The plan is to have your metabolism stoked enough that you will be able to eat twenty-five hundred to three thousand calories a day. You will eat normally (if three thousand calories a day feels normal), weigh in every day, and go back to Phase 1 briefly when and if you notice that you're gaining a few pounds. With this cycling, the diet promises that you will eventually build your metabolism to the point that you can always eat normally if you just go on Phase 1 for two days a month.

Exercise

If you're not into socializing with the whole henhouse while you exercise, then this plan may not be for you. At the Curves centers, you'll exercise on hydraulic machines. Depending on how large the center is, you'll have between eight and twelve machines to choose from. The machines are placed in a circle, with wooden boards between them. You will exercise for thirty-second intervals as hard as you can on a machine. Then a signal will announce that it is time to rotate. Get off your machine and walk in place on the wooden board between machines before getting on the next machine. You'll repeat the entire aerobic and strength-training circuit two to three times, depending on the number of machines the facility has. The goal is to do this thirty-minute workout three days a week.

The Curves at Home workout is also a combination strength-training and cardio workout. In this workout, though, you will alternate strength training via exercise tubes with the cardio of your choice, for forty-second intervals.

The whole plan is very simple and supereasy to follow. At only thirty minutes a day, it seems as though anybody could fit this into her schedule. Surprisingly, though, one of the top reasons our fit chicks left Curves was that they couldn't fit it into their schedule. This may not be just an excuse. Curves does not offer day care, and it generally has limited hours, which was a stumbling block for many of our working women and mothers. But here are a few thoughts from our fit chicks in the Curves program:

Q: Can I go to Curves every day? I read that new government guidelines called for sixty to ninety minutes of exercise a day, but Curves recommends much less—thirty minutes, three times a week.

3FC: Yes, you can go more than the three days a week that Curves recommends, but you should not do the full workout each time. It's easy to assume that if three times a week is good, then five times a week must be even better! But this isn't actually the case. Sometimes, especially when it comes to health, less is more. Your muscles need time to heal between workouts—at least one day of rest between sessions. The book suggests that if you want to go every day, then on alternate days you should work at 50 percent or less of your maximum ability. This means you should just go through the motions on the machines for your light days, and concentrate on a cardio workout, which happens every time you switch machines.

The American Council on Exercise has found that you burn 184 calories during the regular thirty-minute workout at Curves. If you cut down the intensity on your off days at Curves, you will be burning a minimal amount of calories in those sessions. Instead of doing extra days at Curves, consider joining a larger gym with more intense cardio choices, or try supplementing with some cardio videos at home so you'll make the most of your exercise time and burn the calories you need to in order to lose the weight.

Q: I get bored and give up every diet that I try. What makes Curves any different?

3FC: The folks at Curves try very hard to make their workout regimen fun for their members. It may not be as good as a bag of popcorn and *Sex and the City* reruns, but they try. First, they specialize in quick workouts. You only have to stick with it for thirty minutes a day, three times a week. While you are there, you're in a circle facing other members. Regulars get to know each other and look forward to spending time there with their workout buddies. Additionally, the staff usually tries to make it fun. They may play games, give away prizes, or have "brag boards" where they post accomplishments for everyone to read. Activities vary from club to club since franchises are independently owned.

So if you're a chick who loves people but hates to exercise, Curves might be a great choice for you. But not everybody is a social butterfly, so if you don't like to chat and play bingo while you work out, look for another plan. Many of the clubs play music tracks that are made specially for Curves. These are, in general, songs you are familiar with, rerecorded by different artists.

If you try Curves and like it, buy a few months' worth of membership at a time, and you may find you are more committed to the process. Stick with it until you've made exercise a habit. Some people just don't have the discipline to stick to a program at home because they haven't made an investment, and they don't have somebody with a clipboard holding them accountable. We don't recommend going to Curves more than the prescribed three times a week if you are prone to burnout, and we don't recommend buying long-term contracts. While some chicks love it and stick with it for years, some prefer to move on to an exercise regimen that offers more variation.

Q: What kind of food can I have on this diet? I've heard different stories about the fruit—berries only, and others say berries and melon. Does this change if I don't exercise?

3FC: We totally understand your confusion. Many people confuse or mesh this program with other low-carb plans. This plan is completely distinct, however, from any other low-carb plan that is on the market. You can have any food you want as long as you do not exceed the daily carb limit. Some foods will be limited or not allowed based on the daily requirement. For instance, a piece of rhubarb cobbler will have more carbs than are allowed in a day, so you won't be eating one of those. A banana will have a lot of carbs, but if you plan it into your day, you can have it. Nobody is going to gasp if you sprinkle some flour into a sauce, or if you use a splash of teriyaki sauce. As long as you don't exceed your daily carb requirement, you are free to eat what you like.

You can do the Curves diet plan without exercising, but we recommend that you do not count your protein shake as free if you are not doing some sort of strength training. You will probably also have to follow the Calorie Sensitive Plan since you will be burning fewer calories. If you want the full benefits from this plan, you'll have to exercise.

curve balls

The chicks we surveyed had strong opinions about Curves both for and against. Here are the curve balls that made the difference for our Curves chicks between striking out and hitting a home run.

Music Some chicks loved the energizing, upbeat tempo that carried them through the workout. Others had problems with some of the clubs' playing their own line of Christian-based exercise music. Members of other faiths were not comfortable or inspired.

Staff Some chicks felt like family at their Curves. They had involved, dedicated instructors who tried to make their exercise

• *Continued on next page* •

a positive and enjoyable experience. Others were bothered by a lack of exercise and fitness knowledge on the part of the staff.

Facility The small, intimate atmosphere is a big hit with some chicks. Others didn't like the fact that the club didn't have showers or facilities for clients to clean up after exercising on the go.

Results Curves has helped many chicks lose weight who failed in the past. Other chicks who had some experience with other exercise programs felt that Curves was a step back, and they didn't get the results they hoped for.

a day in the food life of a curves chick

This is a sample day on Phase 2, where you will spend most of your time on the Curves program. Be careful, though; your mileage may vary as brands and recipes may have different carb and calorie counts.

Meal 1 • 1 egg scrambled with 2 egg whites, mushrooms, and scallions
Meal 2 • Free shake
Meal 3 • 2 deviled egg halves, turkey sandwich on reduced-carb bread

Meal 4 • Grilled chicken breast, salad with free toppings, plus cherry tomatoes, 1 serving of ranch dressing, steamed green beans
Meal 5 • Tuna salad with ½ cup grapes
Meal 6 • Sugar-free hot cocoa and sugar-free raspberry Jell-O

curves in an eggshell

Professional Counseling The instructors at Curves are there to make sure you do the exercises correctly, and they will help you diagnose problems you might have with your weight loss, but they are generally not trained professionals. The franchise owners complete a training session, and they train the staff.

Support System Curves has a wonderful support system through employees and clientele. The equipment is laid out for strong interaction, and many of the Curves play games or recognize "losers" in some way.

Fitness Factor Curves strongly suggests their signature thirty-minute workouts. However, the exercise doesn't grow with you, and you may hit a fitness standstill when you want to take it to the next level.

Family-Friendly The diet portion is fairly easy to follow if you are cooking for a family. With limited facility hours and no day

● *Continued on next page* ●

care, Curves is much more family-friendly to the employees than to the patrons.

Pros The environment is nonintimidating and can get many women into a regular exercise routine who might not have done it otherwise. The diet is easy to follow, without a lot of fine print.

Cons The workout maxes out early on, not giving much room to take fitness to a higher level, and offers little variety.

$$ Varies from location to location. Memberships can be found as cheaply as $29 per month. Discounts are given if contracts are signed. Beware of high-cost supplements for sale at the facilities. The home workout is inexpensive. The diet portion is average, depending on your taste in protein.

The Person This Diet Is Best For Someone starting out in fitness and open to socializing while exercising. Not everyone wants to be chatting while sweating off the pounds!

recipes from the front lines

JORGE CRUISE: 8 MINUTES IN THE MORNING AND THE 3-HOUR DIET

We lightened our version of muffuletta by replacing some of the olives with diced fresh zucchini squash. As the mixture marinates, the zucchini absorbs all of the salty flavors of the salad, and you'll never know the difference! We chose to pair it with a reduced-fat Swiss and extra-lean ham, leaving out the higher-fat cheeses and meats.

mighty muffuletta

Serves 4

¼ cup chopped onion
¼ cup chopped black olives
¼ cup chopped green olives
½ cup diced zucchini (¼-inch dice)
¼ cup chopped roasted red bell peppers
2 pepperoncini peppers, minced
1 tablespoon olive oil
1 tablespoon red wine vinegar
Few cracks of freshly ground black pepper, to taste
4 ounces extra-lean ham, shaved
2 ounces reduced-fat Swiss cheese, sliced thin
4 whole-wheat pita bread halves, split open

• *Continued on next page* •

In a small mixing bowl, combine onions, olives, zucchini, red bell peppers, pepperoncini, olive oil, vinegar, and black pepper. Cover and chill for several hours or overnight.

To prepare sandwich: Line pita halves with ham and the slices of cheese. Stuff with the olive mixture and enjoy!

Per serving: 192 calories, 7 grams fat, 20 grams carbs, 3 grams fiber, 13 grams protein

You'll find all of the distinctive flavors of Buffalo chicken in our easy salad, and it couldn't be more perfect for a pita.

buffalo chicken salad pita

Serves 6

1 can (12 ounces) chicken breast chunks
1 teaspoon hot sauce
¼ cup light mayonnaise
¼ cup light sour cream
¼ cup crumbled blue cheese
1 stalk celery, finely chopped
½ cup grape tomatoes, cut in half
Freshly cracked black pepper to taste
3 pita rounds, cut in half
1 cup lettuce leaves

Drain canned chicken and add to medium mixing bowl. Sprinkle with hot sauce and toss well; set aside. In small mixing bowl, combine mayonnaise, sour cream, and blue cheese; blend well. Add mayonnaise mixture to chicken and toss to coat. Stir in celery and tomatoes, and add pepper to taste. Line pita halves with a few lettuce leaves, then fill with the chicken salad to serve.

Per serving: 291 calories, 9 grams fat, 28 grams carbs, 3 grams fiber, 22 grams protein

BODY FOR LIFE

Here's a fit chicks fav that makes Body for Life that much tastier. With recipes like this, you won't be longing for Free Day to have dinner with flavor.

shrimp with asparagus and couscous

Serves 4

1 box Near East couscous, Parmesan flavor
1 tablespoon olive oil
1 pound shrimp, peeled and deveined
2 cups asparagus tips
1 medium tomato, diced

Prepare couscous according to package directions. Meanwhile heat olive oil in a nonstick skillet over medium heat. Add asparagus tips and shrimp; stir until shrimp is done. Add chopped tomato and stir briefly to heat through. Combine shrimp mixture with couscous to serve.

Per serving: 309 calories, 8 grams fat, 35 grams carbs, 3 grams fiber, 26 grams protein

BODY FOR LIFE FOR WOMEN

We like to buy frozen chopped spinach in the loose-pack bags and toss a handful into many recipes to sneak in more veggies.

seafood stuffed peppers

Serves 2

1 cup frozen spinach, loose pack
½ cup whole-wheat pasta (dry), tiny shells or elbows
1 teaspoon oil
2 tablespoons finely chopped onion
½ cup low-fat cottage cheese
2 ounces surimi crab, chopped, or use chopped shrimp
1 ounce reduced-fat Swiss cheese, shredded or cut into small
    pieces
Salt and pepper to taste
2 large, sweet red bell peppers, tops and seed core removed

Preheat oven to 350°F. Allow spinach to thaw, then squeeze out moisture. Set aside.

Prepare pasta according to package directions, but remove from water just before done. Pasta will continue to cook in the oven, so you don't want it to get mushy. Drain and place in a medium mixing bowl and set aside.

Meanwhile, heat oil in a nonstick skillet and sauté onion until just translucent. Add thawed and squeezed spinach to skillet and stir to combine. Remove from heat and add to mixing bowl with pasta.

Place cottage cheese in bowl of food processor, and process

until creamy. Combine pasta, seafood, spinach and onions, cottage cheese, Swiss cheese, and salt and pepper to taste. Stuff mixture into bell peppers. Place in a small baking dish and cover with foil. Bake for one hour or until peppers are tender.

Per serving: 262 calories, 5 grams fat, 34 grams carbs, 7 grams fiber, 24 grams protein

Nonstarchy vegetables are allowed almost endlessly. So when you're in the mood for some quantity, try this recipe for a delicious addition to your lean protein choice!

savory roasted green beans

Serves 4

1 bag (16 ounces) frozen whole green beans (do not thaw)
4 teaspoons olive oil
1 tablespoon Worcestershire sauce
Kosher salt to taste
Freshly cracked black pepper (use plenty!)

Preheat oven to 425°F. Toss all ingredients in the bottom of a jelly roll pan, and spread out in single layer. Roast in the oven for 12 to 17 minutes, depending on the thickness of the beans, until they begin to shrivel and become slightly dark.

Per serving: 80 calories, 5 grams fat, 1 gram saturated fat, 9 carbs, 3 grams fiber, 2 grams protein

CURVES

These "free shakes" are free as long as they contain less than twenty carbs and more than twenty grams of protein. So the chicks make them with plain, unflavored protein powder. It's definitely an acquired taste.

apple pie free shake

Serves 1

¼ cup unsweetened applesauce
3 tablespoons nonfat vanilla yogurt, no sugar added
¾ cup skim milk
1 scoop plain, unflavored protein powder (15 g protein per
   scoop)
Hefty dash cinnamon or apple pie spice
2 or 3 ice cubes

Combine all ingredients in a blender and blend until smooth. Pour in a tall glass to serve.

Per serving: 178 calories, 1 gram fat, 20 grams carbs, 1 gram fiber, 23 grams protein

Words to Live By

I often take exercise. Why, only yesterday I had my breakfast in bed.
— OSCAR WILDE

I keep trying to lose weight . . . but it keeps finding me!
— AUTHOR UNKNOWN

chicks in the zone
the zone diet

I F YOU'RE INTO losing weight while maintaining a round-the-clock natural high that makes taking the pounds off painless, then the Zone diet from Dr. Barry Sears may be a plan that will work for you. In essence, the Zone is a well-balanced diet plan that restricts starchy carbs, which, admittedly, are the only carbs worth talking about for many of us. However, rather than just cutting out carbs, the Zone emphasizes a perfect balance of protein, fat, and carbs. This plan is roughly 40 percent protein, 30 percent carbs, and 30 percent fat.

The Zone is commonly referred to as a low-carb diet, which seems to be a real pet peeve of Dr. Sears. And comparing it to traditional low-carb diets, we would have to agree that it isn't just a fancy version of Atkins, but it could still be considered a *reduced*-carb diet. The National Institutes of Health considers the average diet to be 45 to 65 percent carbohydrates. At 30 percent carbs, this plan is at about the third rung on the low-carb limbo stick, not the floor-rubbing bottom rung that Atkins chicks play at.

Before you run out to stock up on corn on the cob and crescent rolls to go with your rib-eye steak, take a minute to read the fine print. The Zone plan calls for mostly lean protein and nonstarchy carbs, like grilled chicken, steamed green beans, bowls of fruit, and other foods that won't heavily impact your glucose levels.

If you manage to maintain this nutritional balance, Dr. Sears tells us, you will enter a state of hormonal bliss called "the Zone." The Zone is a physical state of harmony that we achieve when we maintain the correct level of insulin (affectionately known as the fat storage hormone), in our bloodstreams.

Dr. Sears claims that if you can keep your insulin from becoming either too high or too low, you will not only lose weight without being hungry, but your health and overall sense of well-being will be drastically improved and you will achieve something called "SuperHealth." Who could ask for anything more?

One easy way to enter the Zone and stay there: before each meal, you must mentally divide your plate into three equal sections. In one section you will have a portion of lean protein. Then you will fill up the rest of the plate with Zone-friendly veggies and fruit, with a dab of good fat, like olive oil, or almond slices. You'll do this for three meals a day.

For snacks, you will follow the same ratio, but with a smaller plate. How much you are allowed to put on your plate depends on your activity level and your lean body mass, which Dr. Sears teaches you how to calculate. This is called your "protein prescription."

The alternate method to counting on the Zone diet is relatively easy to master. You'll be eating a prescribed number of "blocks," depending on your body composition and activity level. The average woman will get three block meals a day. At each meal you can have three blocks each of protein, carbs, and fat. A block of protein is generally equal to an ounce of lean protein. A block of carbs can range from several cups of chopped spinach to one-third cup of mashed potatoes. Clearly, the more advance planning you do, the more bang you can get for your Zone buck. There are numerous books on the Zone, including *Zone Blocks*, which has lists of block portions for every kind of food imaginable. If you want bacon and eggs for breakfast, you can look it up in the book and see, for instance, that two egg whites equal a block, and so does one whole egg or three slices of turkey bacon. If, like most women, you eat three blocks per meal, you can have, for example, nine slices of turkey bacon or six egg whites or any other three-block calculation of protein at your meal. While you're at it, you can look up your fats and carbs and round out your whole plate, Zone style.

While it may sound easy enough to look up your foods and pick individual ingredients, it isn't always easy to make an actual recipe. The majority of your family recipes are not going to be Zone ready, and many just can't be converted at all. It's not much fun to pick apart your meal to try to come out with the correct portions. You'll find it much easier to stick to Zone recipes.

Are you still with us? Now comes the hard part—which is to say, the carbohydrate part. The Zone recommends very few grains; most of your carbohydrates will come in the form of low-density carbs like broccoli, cauliflower, cabbage, or greens. Bread, pasta, and rice should be eaten sparingly, much like a garnish. Grains are high in calories and carbohydrates, and they also have a high impact on insulin, which is the enemy of SuperHealth.

According to Dr. Sears, though, all those starchy carbohydrates like mashed potatoes and cinnamon rolls won't be hard to give up, because within a few days you will enter the Zone, where there is no such thing as a Big Mac attack, and Krispy Kreme doughnuts will never again whisper to you across a crowded room.

Dr. Sears contends that by keeping your insulin in balance, you will be able to lose weight and keep it off. To maintain this balance, you need to eat at regular intervals. You will be eating up to five times a day. While the diet is essentially a low-calorie diet, you can eat a large volume of food, so you shouldn't get hungry. You can access more Zone resources and read more examples of food combinations at www.3fatchicks.com/thezone.

So is there really a magical place called SuperHealth where you can give up cookies and cakes and cream puffs and lose weight without even a twinge of a craving? Well, that depends upon whom you ask.

When the Zone was at its peak in popularity back in the nineties, we didn't give it much of a chance. For us, it was too much of a hassle to tabulate 40 percent protein, 30 percent carbs, and 30 percent fat. It seemed like a diet for mathletes. Also, while it's a wonderful idea to get your body into a hormonal state that will give you superhealth and allow you to lose weight painlessly, we're not entirely sure that any of those claims are true. We're not scientists and we don't know of any independent research done on this question other than by the Zone folks. We do know that the calculations are ridiculously thought-intensive for meal planning, and we're not too sure we'd ever be happy with three ounces of chicken, three cups of green beans, and a sprinkle of almonds at mealtime. Also, the strict balance of foods that needs to be adhered to on this diet can be difficult. You could potentially have to eat a whole package of tofu and thirty-six spears of asparagus for dinner to balance the six cashews you nibbled while you were cooking, or risk falling out of the Zone. And all measurements have to be precise; one teaspoon too much of this ingredient or the other could damage your biochemical euphoria. Trying to make recipes that actually mesh well is even harder, so this is a good diet if you are somebody who is happy with simple mixes and combinations. But for most of us, eating in the Zone can get a little boring.

We never personally knew anybody on the Zone, but obviously, this diet has worked for a lot of people out there, so we recently asked our on-line chicks in the Zone what they thought about Barry Sears's plan, and here are some of the questions and comments that they shared.

meet the chicks in the zone

Marion from California

I've tried a few diets but never stayed on them because I hate to cook and I hate most frozen dinners. What else was left but restaurants! I heard about local delivery of fresh Zone meals. They cook a meal fresh and bring it right to you. It's almost like having my own personal chef.

And since portions are controlled, I can't overeat. It's pricey, but it's worth it. I don't think I've ever been so excited about losing weight!

Sarah from Colorado
I finally broke my plateau since starting the Zone! I weighed in at 139 pounds this morning—the first time I have been below 140 pounds in well over a year! This is so exciting! I think completely giving up rice, pasta, and bread gave me the extra "shove" I needed to break through. For the past week, I have been getting all of my carbs from fruits and veggies, and I'm not the least bit hungry.

Rachel from Florida
I've been counting calories for a few weeks and just recently decided to eat fewer carbs and more protein. So I tweaked my plan a little and it turns out that I had adjusted it close to a 40/30/30 ratio, which I remembered from a Zone book I had read a while back. I pulled the book back out and reread it, and now I'm hooked! The plan makes so much sense and it's so much easier than all the extreme low-carb plans. The Zone seems like just the right amount of everything.

Sue from Tennessee
My husband has been packing on the pounds lately. I don't need to lose weight, but I've been preparing Zone meals for both of us. I don't think he even realizes it, and I haven't told him. We've been eating healthier foods like chicken and salmon. I finally asked him to weigh himself, and he's lost seven pounds so far!

Q: I am hardly losing weight. I'm eating the correct blocks of food and exercising every day, but I'm only losing about half a pound per week. What am I doing wrong?

3FC: You're not doing anything wrong. The Zone does not produce quick results. This is not a thin-thighs-in-thirty-days program. The Zone is a fat-burning diet, and therefore you don't drop quick water weight or lean muscle tissue as on the Atkins diet. You should be losing weight at the rate of no more than one to one and a half pounds per week. Depending on how much you have to lose, you may already be losing weight at a very reasonable rate.

You may want to double-check your lean body mass. It's possible that your lean body mass is rising, which means you are losing fat but gaining lean muscle tissue, which in turn can make you heavier, even though you are looking and feeling more fit. Look at the big picture and don't rely on the scale. Your tape measure should show some results.

If not, look again at the rules of the plan. Are you drinking enough water? Are you measuring your food, or trying to eyeball the portion sizes? Maybe your eyes are bigger than your portion restrictions. Read *The Zone* again to refresh your memory, and make double sure that you are counting your blocks correctly. Not all carbs are created equal. For instance, one block of strawberries is equal to one-third cup of oatmeal.

One more thing you can try—revisit your activity level categories. This may also be a good time to check your exercise level and see if you can add anything to your program. And don't forget to leave enough time between meals so that you can keep your insulin steady and stay in the Zone.

To Market, to Market

If you're taking it on the lam, it's a good idea to bring along some emergency rations so that you can stay in the Zone even though you're away from home. Here are some ideas for what to pack in your brown bag. Mix and match as necessary to make a Zone-ready meal or snack.

1. Tuna or chicken in pouches or tins
2. Reduced-fat cheese sticks

3. Ready-to-drink shakes
4. Protein shake mix and canned milk
5. Applesauce cups
6. An orange or other fresh fruit
7. Chopped raw veggies, like cucumber and broccoli, with cherry tomatoes
8. Almonds and peanuts
9. Hershey SmartZone bars
10. Cash for a fast-food grilled chicken salad

Q: All I ever eat for breakfast are egg white omelets, and I can't take another one. Any suggestions, besides sleeping until lunch?

3FC: You're in luck. Although egg whites are optimal choices, they can get old quick. So break a few rules that won't cost you calories, and have lunch for breakfast. Try eating our salad on page 192, protein-fortified pudding, cottage cheese and fruit, or even a meal replacement shake, such as a ready-to-drink ZonePerfect shake. There are Zone-authorized meals and snacks available; you'll find a current list at www.3fatchicks.com/thezone.

If you prefer strictly breakfast foods for breakfast, you might try making a quiche—chock-full of vegetables—or boiled eggs, protein pancakes, crepes, or even oatmeal and turkey bacon. Try to incorporate fresh fruit into your meal for a more invigorating breakfast. A meal of almond-sprinkled oatmeal, strawberries, and scrambled egg substitute is right on target.

Q: I'm confused. I thought bananas were okay, but now I've heard they are unfavorable carbs. Am I not supposed to be eating them? I'm not sure I can do without my banana in the morning.

3FC: You can eat unfavorable carbs, which unfortunately include bananas, but it is best that you limit them as much as you can. Keep unfavorable carbs to 25 percent of your total carb intake. This means if you get four blocks per meal, one of your blocks can be an unfavorable carb. However, if you have a three-block meal, that's a little harder to calculate! You'll be able to eat more food if you restrict unfavorable carbs, and you won't risk falling out of the Zone because of fluctuating insulin levels.

So the answer is yes, you can enjoy a banana every now and again, but you should try to eat fewer of them, which can be hard at first, we know. As you get used to the program and enjoy the feeling of Super-Health, you'll be happier doing without the foods you currently crave. In fact, Dr. Sears recommends eating a carb-rich meal once a month. This is so the carb hangover will remind you how being out of the Zone feels. This lesson will both help keep you focused and give you a chance to enjoy the foods you miss!

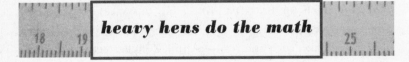

heavy hens do the math

We asked our heavy hens to crunch their numbers, and here are some of the sobering figures they came up with.

- 67 percent were overweight as children.
- 84 percent have immediate family members who are also overweight.
- 32 percent have been on more than twenty diets.
- 80 percent have *not* been diagnosed with a health condition that affected their weight.
- 87 percent felt lack of motivation because their goal weights were so far away and did not seem attainable.

- 20 percent said they walk for exercise because it is easier for them than other activities.
- 21 percent had joined a gym.
- 12 percent were not able to exercise yet, because of their size.
- Only 8 percent felt embarrassed to exercise in front of others. The rest exercise in various ways at home.
- 24 percent said the fear of sagging, excess skin deterred them from losing weight.

Q: I am able to stick to this plan really well, but I'm having a problem on the weekends when I'm off work. I get wild snack attacks, and I occasionally give in. It's just so difficult sometimes!

3FC: If you are truly in the Zone, a hormonal state that lasts around the clock, you should not be experiencing hunger. You may experience difficulties if you spread your meals too far apart or if you are eating the incorrect volumes or ratios. Double-check your weekend food against the acceptable food list, and make sure you are eating meals or snacks no more than five hours apart.

If you're sure that you're eating correctly, your problem may be a case of head hunger. It's fairly common for people to reach for food when stressed, tired, or anxious. It might help to switch the order of your meals and snacks. Try a protein shake for your next meal. It will be balanced and sweet enough that, hopefully, your cravings will subside.

Q: I'm interested in lower-carb diets, but I'm a vegetarian. I tried Atkins once and it was a disaster. Can I do the Zone without eating a block of tofu for every meal? My regular diet is primarily grains, veggie burgers, and tofu.

3FC: The Zone is very soy-friendly. Dr. Sears says that the vegetarian version may even be the healthiest version available. You can have tofu, soy meat substitutes, eggs, and some dairy products to fill your portion of daily protein.

It is easier to be a vegetarian on the Zone than it is on Atkins. On Atkins, you eat mostly protein and fat, with a much smaller portion of vegetables. That doesn't leave a lot of choices for a vegetarian. On the Zone, you eat lower fat, with a much closer ratio of carbs and protein. This means you can have plenty of vegetables on your plate and even some grains once in a while, not just a brick of tofu.

Q: I'm having problems with constipation. If I take fiber supplements, do I have to count them as carb blocks? I'd rather eat my carbs than dissolve them in a glass of water.

3FC: Fiber supplements do not count as carbohydrate blocks as long as they are just straight fiber. "Fiber cookies" would count as a carb, as they also have flour and sugar. Dr. Sears says he first used the phrase "net carbs" in 1995 for calculating carbs. His definition of net carbs is carbohydrates minus fiber, and that is what should be counted for your carb block. When the low carb-craze hit, the phrase "net carbs for Atkins" became very popular; it also included subtracting sugar alcohols from the total. On the Zone, you will subtract only fiber. So, as long as your fiber is straight fiber, you are free to use it. You should also try to incorporate more fiber into your diet so you will not need to use supplements.

Q: There is so much technical information in the book, and honestly, I just don't get it. How do the blocks work, simply speaking? I can't stick to this plan if I have to struggle to plan a meal.

3FC: Originally, meals were described as comprising 40 percent protein, 30 percent carbohydrates, and 30 percent fat. This was just a general idea; it has been refined over the years. An updated version of this formula is the block method. This way of counting will save you from having to carry a nutritional guide and a calculator to the dinner table.

Each meal is divided into Zone blocks. The number of blocks you get to eat is based on factors such as your activity level. Blocks consist of mini-blocks for each group of fat, carbs, and protein. For example, if you get to eat three blocks at mealtime, you'll have three blocks of protein, three blocks of carbs, and three blocks of fat. If you get one block at snack time, that means one block of protein, one block of carbohydrates, and one block of fat.

You must always include all three groups. Portion size depends on the type of food you choose. A block of protein equals one ounce of lean meat. Some protein blocks give you larger portions, like two ounces of shrimp. Carbohydrates vary widely, from several cups of chopped spinach, to a quarter cup of pasta. Fats range from one-third of a teaspoon for oils to six peanuts. You can mix and match from the lists to build your perfect Zone meal.

Complete lists of the portions are included on the Zone Web site and in recent Zone books, such as *Mastering the Zone, The Top 100 Zone Foods,* and *What to Eat in the Zone.*

Dr. Sears actually recommends eyeballing the portions. He says to eat a palm-sized portion of meat, which will take up one-third of your plate. You can fill up the rest of the plate with nonstarchy vegetables and add a splash of good fat. We have to admit it sounds easier than it is. We're not sure how eyeballing the portion sizes can be that helpful if it takes just the right balance to enter the Zone. When portions such as one-third teaspoon oil are involved, or carbohydrate portions that vary from one-third cup peas to four cups cucumbers, it just seems smarter to have a handbook and some measuring spoons handy.

Q: I'm thinking about leaving my low-carb diet and entering the Zone. Am I still going to lose weight? I've lost twenty pounds on low-carb, but I'm ready for some more variety.

3FC: If you are on a strict low-carb diet, then you may very well gain a few pounds as you reintroduce carbs. This isn't fat, however. You'll be regaining water weight you lost at the start of your low-carb diet. Relax, it will come off again on the Zone, only this time you should be losing fat instead of just water!

Q: The Zone recommends fish oil every day. Can I use something else, like flaxseed oil? The fish oil capsules are huge, and sometimes I burp fish through the day.

3FC: The fish oil has been chosen not just for the omega-3 oils but also for the essential acids EPA and DHA. Taking other oils might be helpful, but not as effective for the purposes that Dr. Sears has outlined in his book.

If you can't take a large capsule, you can burst the capsules and take the liquid straight, or mix it in with cottage cheese or a nutritional shake—not a very appetizing thought. You can also look for smaller capsules and increase the number of capsules you take to reach the dose you need.

If you haven't taken fish oil recently, you might be happy to know that there are newer brands on the market that may not give you indigestion. They are more expensive, but they are purer, and will have fewer side effects. Look for an ultrarefined fish oil, commonly advertised as having "no fishy aftertaste." Mmm, what more could a girl ask for? You can also explore vegetarian supplement options at your local health food store.

We would like to note that you should not take fish oil supplements without speaking to your doctor first. Fish oil can interact with and worsen the effects of certain medications or medical conditions.

the zone in an eggshell

Professional Counseling None.

Support System There is a forum at the official site and various forums across the Internet.

Fitness Factor There is no official guideline for exercise, but the amount of food you eat is based on your activity level.

Family-Friendly You can feed the whole family on Zone foods. All you have to do is measure out your own portions.

Pros Wholesome foods and a balanced diet. You're less likely to get hungry on this plan than on plans like the South Beach diet.

Cons Very few convenience foods. Might be monotonous for the traveler because of the lack of fast-food options. Measuring can be tedious until you get skilled at eyeballing portions. Non-Zone recipes with multiple ingredients can be hard to convert to Zone portions.

$$ Can be somewhat expensive with more meat and veggies; however, the reduction in junk food helps to compensate, so you probably won't notice a difference in your budget.

The Person This Diet Is Best For Somebody who doesn't mind measuring and having specific guidelines on how to eat. Also vegetarians.

recipes from the front lines

This untraditional breakfast is a great way to get out of the "I'm bored with breakfast" blues. You should note that this recipe does include the unfavorable carb maple syrup. Keep an eye on your unfavorable carb list, and don't overindulge too often.

"i'm bored with breakfast" salad

Serves 1

3 cups spring mix, or other leafy lettuce
3 slices turkey bacon, cooked and torn in bite-sized pieces
½ teaspoon canola oil
½ teaspoon red wine vinegar
½ teaspoon Dijon mustard
¼ teaspoon coarsely ground black pepper
4 teaspoons reduced-sugar maple syrup
Cooking spray
1 egg plus 2 egg whites

Place lettuce mixture in salad bowl and mix with turkey bacon. Set aside. In small bowl, add oil, vinegar, mustard, pepper, and syrup. Mix thoroughly and drizzle over the lettuce and bacon mixture. Toss to cover all the lettuce and bacon.

Spray warm skillet with cooking spray and add the whole

egg and egg whites. Puncture yolk so it spreads across egg whites. When egg sets, turn over and cook the other side. When egg is completely cooked, chop into bite-sized pieces with the edge of the egg turner. Pour chopped egg onto salad mixture and serve immediately.

Per serving: 314 calories, 15 grams fat, 24 grams carbs, 2 grams fiber, 21 grams protein

---

Here's a recipe that keeps the precious balance you need in order to stay in the Zone!

chicken cashew stir fry

* * * * * * * * * * * * * * * * *

Serves 1

1½ teaspoons soy sauce
1 teaspoon cornstarch (1 carb block)
1 teaspoon broth or cold water
½ cup nonfat chicken broth
3 ounces chicken breast, skinless, cut into thin strips (3 protein blocks)
¼ teaspoon freshly grated ginger
1 clove garlic, minced
½ cup broccoli, cut up (⅓ carb block)
1 red bell pepper, cored and chopped (⅓ carb block)
½ cup sliced onion (⅓ carb block)
⅓ cup sliced water chestnuts (1 carb block)
9 whole cashews, split in half (3 fat blocks)

● *Continued on next page* ●

In a small bowl, combine soy sauce, cornstarch, and water or broth. Stir until smooth and set aside.

Heat ¼ cup of the chicken broth in a nonstick skillet over medium high heat, and add chicken strips, garlic, and ginger. Stir for a couple of minutes until chicken is done. Add remaining ¼-cup broth, the vegetables, and cashews, and continue to stir and cook until crisp tender, or to the degree of doneness that you prefer. Add reserved cornstarch mixture and stir quickly until all is coated and sauce is slightly thickened.

Words to Live By

My whole life, I've wanted to feel comfortable in my skin. It's the most liberating thing in the world. — DREW BARRYMORE

Avoid any diet that discourages the use of hot fudge.
—DON KARDONG

8

grand ole oprah chicks

bob greene, oprah's boot camp, dr. phil

FROM THE THIGH MASTER to the Ab Roller to Trimspa Baby! we fat chicks are fascinated with celebrity fitness products, plans, and endorsements. We rush out in droves to buy the latest craze, convinced that after only ten minutes each day, we too can have thighs, buns, and six-pack abs like the stars. Unfortunately, most of us discover that our celebrity fitness miracle is a more useful clothes hanger than a makeover machine. But in the world of Tinseltown trim-downs, there is one role model who for us is worth her weight in gold.

Oprah is the be-all and end-all of weight-loss queens. When Oprah lost weight, we cheered and we loved her, and were never jealous. When she gained weight, we felt her pain, and we understood, because we had been there. When Oprah climbed back up on the diet horse, we hung on to every pound through every episode. We chatted about how chiseled her cheekbones looked, how her hips were getting smaller, and how tiny her waistline had become. When she wheeled out the wagon o' fat to show how much weight she had lost, flashing her skinny jeans to the cameras, we vowed to pass the story down to our children and their children, for years to come. Meanwhile, Calvin Klein jeans flew off the shelves all over the planet.

Looking at the competition, nobody else comes close to being our weight-loss guru. Suzanne Somers, the trim, perky pigtailed blonde who kept us company throughout the seventies, struggled to lose a mere fifteen pounds, but it was lost and documented before we ever knew it happened. Marilu Henner lost around fifty pounds and invested more blood, sweat, and tears in her weight-loss process, but she wasn't in our living rooms every afternoon loving us like Oprah was. And Anna "Trimspa, Baby!" Nicole Smith, well . . . we'll let Anna speak for herself.

So why has Oprah been able to influence hundreds of thousands, if not millions, of us fat chicks to actually do something about our health? After all, she isn't really just one of the girls. The woman is a gazillionaire. Oprah has mansions, trainers, personal gyms, assistants, maids, cooks, and chauffeurs. She can pay someone to lift her legs, cook her meals, and then wipe her brow when she's done. Oprah is one of the most powerful people in America, and definitely one of the richest. So why does Oprah inspire us to lose weight, even though she obviously has a whole lot more help reaching her goal than we ever will?

Well, because Oprah lets us take a peek at the real struggle of weight loss. Oprah took responsibility for every bite that went in her mouth, and she didn't try to make the process look simple or slick. She wanted french fries, damn it, and we understood! She resisted exercise, got frustrated, and told us about where she was going wrong. She shared her bad experiences as well as her joys, and women all over the country who had ridden the same roller-coaster fell in love with her.

We also fell in love with her trainers. Bob Greene became a fitness guru because he and his Make the Connection program helped Oprah get in shape. We 3 fat chicks bought the "Make the Connection" video and all piled up together and watched it from beginning to end, armed with a box of Kleenex. From that day forward, we got together for Fat Chick Day once a week. This was a day we devoted to our futures. We discussed diet and exercise and talked about what we really wanted to do for our health. We each bought copies of Bob's book and journal, and we followed his tips and lost weight, just so we could follow in Oprah's footsteps.

We also fell in love with Dr. Phil, who helped Oprah triumph in her infamous Texas beef court battle. And although he was not connected to the fitness world at that time, it was enough for us that he got Oprah into the right mind-set to triumph over all those angry Texans. He taught Oprah how to put mind over meat, and so it was inevitable that Dr. Phil would eventually adapt his pull-yourself-up-by-your-bootstraps approach to life to the weight-loss world. Now chicks from sea to shining sea are chanting his Seven Keys to Weight Loss Freedom, and counting down their dress sizes too, we hope.

Oprah plays a big role in our personal diet histories. She was a celebrity who had the courage to let us know that she was no different from the rest of us. Oprah got fat just like us, lost weight with difficulty just like us, and put the weight back on afterward—*just like us*. But along the way she taught us that if we don't give up, we can achieve our goals. She reminded us that two steps forward and one step back is better than no steps forward at all. Oprah helped us understand that while the battle of the bulge never really ends, if we hold our ground and keep charging up over that hill, we really can trade our potbelly for a pot of gold at the end of our personal rainbow.

So in a book where we have tried to take a look beneath the surface glimmer of diet and fitness plans, and shy away from celebrity, we felt it was important to include the one school of celebrity fitness thinking that really has made a difference to the waistlines of the world.

meet the grand ole oprah chicks

Megan from Kentucky

I could have never lost weight without Oprah. I tried so many diets, and I always failed. Oprah put aside her vanity and she showed us sweat, and she showed us determination, and she showed us victory. I never see celebrities struggle; they hide it from us—but not Oprah. She's got the same weaknesses that we all do, but thanks to her I know that just because I have a weak side, it doesn't mean that I'm not strong. I am strong, I fought the battle, and I won. Thank you, Oprah, for helping me get my life back.

Kery from France

I am a twenty-six-year-old graphic designer. I've had this problem with "bad foods" for a long, long time. I didn't crave vegetables and fruits, but I could go a whole week eating pizza, potatoes, pasta, fast food, cookies, and other junky stuff without even blinking. What caused me to really think about it and make the decision to lose weight was partly reading Dr. Phil McGraw's book; it may seem like "only a book," but it spoke to me in a way that no friend or family member had ever done, and helped me think and understand why I had many "bad" food behaviors—as well as giving me ideas about how to correct them. Granted, it's not a fairy tale, and it's not easy every day. It's been two months now. I wouldn't say it's a struggle for me; it's more like getting slowly accustomed, and once I am, things seem easier and more pleasant.

Keli from Pennsylvania

I recently read the Bob Greene Total Body Makeover. I've read these types of books before but mostly skimmed over parts, and actually doing them was hit or miss. I really read the first chapter on "building a solid emotional foundation." I started looking at why weight loss worked in the past and why it got away from me. I lost sixty-five pounds on Weight Watchers years ago and gained it all back. Bob Greene's concept of "conscious eat-ing," which is really paying attention to what you're eating and why, is helping me. I'm trying to eat for nutrition now, and not for comfort. It's amazing how many times, especially at work, I would eat something that was offered just because it was offered and without even thinking. I found the book enlightening. In fact I'm going to read it again.

BOB GREENE MAKES THE CONNECTION

Oprah's trainer Bob Greene first brought his program to the world when he published his first book, *Make the Connection,* in 1996. Few weight-loss books have been as moving or as willing to bring a new at-titude and approach to weight loss. The central idea was a simple one: if Oprah could do it, we could too.

Make the Connection started the whole Oprah/diet movement. It was a book, video, and companion journal all wrapped up tightly so that even mere mortals like us could lose weight the same way that Oprah did. The book, written by Bob and Oprah, sold millions of copies, and we wish we knew just how many pounds of fat were lost around the world because of it.

Make the Connection was popular not just because of Oprah but also because it was a sound, reasonable approach to weight loss that didn't include a fad diet. The book is still available on Amazon, though the video can only be found on eBay now.

Make the Connection is a multistep approach to weight loss. Here are the steps:

- Do aerobic exercise five to seven days a week, at least twenty to sixty minutes each session.
- Eat three meals and two snacks daily, consisting of a low-fat, balanced diet. Include at least two fruits and three vegetables each day.

- Limit or eliminate alcohol, and drink six to eight glasses of water daily.
- Stop eating two to three hours before bedtime.
- Renew your commitment to a healthy lifestyle each day.

Simple, right? So simple, in fact, that we don't understand why this program isn't still as popular as it was when it first came out. It makes sense, it's easy to follow, and it works. We have even found that our own diet efforts have been more successful when we incorporated these guidelines. But sometimes a chick just needs more. And when we needed more, Bob gave it to us in his second book, *The Total Body Makeover.*

The Total Body Makeover takes a different approach to weight loss and has a stronger focus on exercise than diet. In *Make the Connection,* we did aerobics five to seven times a week. This time Bob added weight training and other exercises for a more complete body work-out. The goal is not just to burn off the fat but to tone up the muscles as well so we can look buff in our workout gear!

The most interesting part of *The Total Body Makeover* is that we are advised not to go on a diet, other than to follow a few basic eating guidelines. We should eat three meals and two snacks every day, and we should never skip breakfast. In fact, Bob puts as much emphasis on starting each day with a nutritious breakfast as Mom did! You should also end each day on the right note. Pick a cutoff point and never eat past that time, period. This one tip has helped many chicks lose a few pounds. The food we eat at night isn't metabolized any differently; it's our food choices late at night that are the true culprit. How many of us pig out on celery sticks while watching Letterman? We're more likely to eat chips or ice cream late at night. Remove the option to eat, and you eliminate the bad foods. It really is a lot easier than it sounds.

In *Make the Connection,* we were advised to go on a low-fat diet. In *The Total Body Makeover,* Bob tells us it is in our best interest not to cut calories too much and to give exercise a chance to help us lose weight first. Don't get too excited just yet. We still have to follow common-sense rules at the kitchen table. A nutritious breakfast doesn't include honey buns or anything floating in gravy. However, you won't have to cut out bread, count points, or refer to a forbidden foods list. If you don't feel comfortable with your progress after the first twelve-week round, then you can go on a more structured, formal diet. What diet would you follow? Any one you want. Bob includes a basic rundown of all the popular diets, from Atkins to Weight Watchers, and invites you to choose the one you like best. Or don't follow a diet at all, just eat healthier foods and don't pig out. If you think that this sounds like the perfect program for the chick who hates to diet but loves to exercise, you would be right! Here are the plan basics:

Total Body Makeover Plan Basics

Five Simple Eating Rules

- Have an eating cutoff time.
- Eat a nourishing breakfast.
- Drink at least six 8-ounce glasses of water each day.
- Eliminate alcohol.
- Make eating a conscious act (eat for the right reasons).

Twelve-Week Exercise Plan

- Functional exercises six times per week
- Strength-training exercises three times per week
- Aerobic exercise five days per week
- Double aerobic exercise on sixth day each week
- Rest on seventh day

Bob Greene has routines for beginning, intermediate, and advanced levels, so you can jump in wherever feels right. The program grows with you, as you graduate to each new level. The total beginner will have no trouble getting started. A good half of the book is just photos of exercises and a twelve-week chart so you know exactly what to do on which days. Bob calls this Boot Camp, and for good reason. It is an intensive exercise program, and you will have to be devoted and work hard. The payoff, though, will be more energy, long-term weight loss, and buns of steel. If you need a little inspiration, we recommend that you rent a copy of *G.I. Jane* and envision yourself as Demi Moore in training.

Whether you choose the original *Make the Connection* or the newer *Total Body Makeover*, you are going to exercise a lot every day, including doing cardio and weights. A lot of people are going to do well with this plan, because you see results right away, which is a great motivator. Besides, we are getting to the point in society where everything goes to extremes, fitness included, so there are a lot of fitness plans out there that are more extreme than these. But the *Total Body Makeover* is going to take more dedication than the other fitness and diet programs we've reviewed in this book. We think that *Make the Connection* takes a slightly gentler approach, even though it requires just as much dedication. It is easy to follow, makes a lot of sense, and could be applied to anyone's life, no matter how much or how little time someone has to devote to a fitness plan. To get a more rounded picture of this program, we asked our Oprah chicks to air in with some of their questions and concerns.

Q: The word aerobics *gives me traumatic flashbacks to the eighties, and I get visions of pink tights and frantic dance movements in time to the sound-track of* Footloose. *Can I do this program without reliving these unpleasant memories?*

3FC: Aerobics does not necessarily equal doing Kevin Bacon–inspired buck-and-wings dressed in a spandex bodysuit. The term covers a wide range of activities, from running to spinning, or even in-line skating. You can choose the activities that you enjoy the most. In fact, you should choose several aerobic activities so you don't get burned out. Variety keeps your exercise routine interesting every day, and you'll be more motivated to continue. Most of the activities are free and can be done in the privacy of your own home. If you do feel a little footloose, you are still free to head to your nearest fitness center and sign up for a dance aerobics class.

Q: There's no way I can eat breakfast every day. I'm not hungry, I don't have time, and I don't even like breakfast food. Can't I just get a big snack later?

3FC: Isn't it funny how breakfast can elicit opposite reactions from people? Some people can't even open their eyes in the morning unless their heads are hovering over a plate of flapjacks, grits, and sausage. Other people consider breakfast a burden and the most expendable of meals. We're told time and time again that if we aren't hungry, just don't eat. This rule doesn't apply at breakfast. Even if you do not feel hungry, have something light, such as our Tomato Basil Eggs on page 218. You'll be less likely to overeat later too. Breakfast doesn't have to include eggs or other traditional foods. Pick a food you really like, so you'll enjoy it. Try a sandwich or a smoothie or a high-protein pizza, such as the frozen South Beach diet pizzas. They are all quick solutions and the beginning of a good habit.

Q: I'm a habitual late-night muncher. I can't watch TV unless I'm eating or go to sleep without a snack. Sometimes I sneak and nibble after the family has gone to bed. I've tried establishing a cutoff time for eating, but I keep slipping back into my habit, and sometimes I "forget" about it. What can I do?

3FC: Late-night munching is a very common problem. Sometimes we eat out of boredom or habit, but rarely out of true hunger. Make a deliberate, conscious effort to break this habit. Set an alarm clock for your cutoff time, so you have a loud reminder to stop eating. Don't rely on your memory if you have the convenient ability to lose track of the time. If necessary, enlist the help of a friend or family member to remind you that your eating day has finished. It won't take long before it feels natural to you.

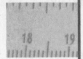

beating the midnight munchies

There's an old saying that idle hands are the devil's tools—definitely true when it comes to late-night snacking. If we can stay busy, we are less likely to slip our hands into the cookie jar. Here are some ideas our chicks shared to help avoid late-night nibbling.

Buy yourself a nice manicure set so you can pamper your fingers at night. You'd never dream of interrupting the polishing and buffing to muss them up with cheese doodle dust! Pedicures are also a good deterrent. You don't want to slide around on the kitchen floor with wet tootsies, so a good soak and shine can help keep you in one place. — DOREEN

Fill your magazine stand with fitness magazines. When the urge hits to reach for a snack, grab a magazine and remind yourself what your goals are. — MARYBETH

Read anything. No, wait, read about sex. Better yet, have sex! — LAURA

Before you reach your eating cutoff time, make sure you take the time to thoroughly enjoy your last snack or meal. It's easy to get distracted and finish your food without noticing a bite, and then you are left craving more food even if you are not physically hungry. Sit down at your table and eat off a pretty dish. Get rid of any distractions, and just savor the moment. You'll find it so satisfying that you probably won't want anything else later. — ANDREA

Let your cell phone help curb nighttime snacking. Take advantage of the free nighttime calls and phone your diet buddies around the country! This is much better than eating! —JACQUELINE

Use teeth-whitening strips at night, to brighten your smile. You can't eat while using them, and you won't want to eat afterwards! —CATHY

Instead of food, try a gourmet tea from vendors such as www.adagio.com. It's flavorful, comforting, and calorie-free, and some people think green tea can even help with weight loss. —DIANA

make the connection in an eggshell

Professional counseling None.

Support System None.

Fitness Factor Regular aerobic exercise is required almost daily.

Family-Friendly Very. You do not have to buy special diet foods, just need to make lower-fat versions of your usual, balanced meals.

Pros Guidelines are very clear and make it easy to stay focused. A companion journal helps you to keep track.

Cons Not as much emphasis on overall fitness as in *The Total Body Makeover.*

● *Continued on next page* ●

$$ Just the cost of the book and the optional companion journal.

The Person This Diet Is Best For Someone who is dedicated, likes a low-fat diet, is willing to exercise daily, and likes having her routine spelled out for her.

---

total body makeover in an eggshell

Professional Counseling None.

Support System Bob offers a support forum on his Web site, www.getwiththeprogram.org, but it is limited and slow, and there doesn't seem to be any official interaction. This program is also supported at eDiets, for a small subscription fee.

Fitness Factor It's all about the fitness. Expect to be dedicated six days a week for this intensive workout program.

Family-Friendly Yes! You are not on a diet with this plan, so you can feed your family your usual meals and not feel left out. If you do opt to diet, your plan will be as family-friendly as the diet you choose.

Pros You don't have to go on a diet plan, just focus on the exercise. It's flexible enough for any fitness level. The book goes into great detail to make sure you understand the exercises and routines.

Cons Some people may have difficulty adapting their lifestyle to this plan, especially if they don't like to eat breakfast or have trouble with the eating cutoff time. It can be hard to fit in all the exercise.

$$ Very affordable! You may need to purchase dumbbells or good walking shoes. You can choose aerobic activities that are not free, such as spinning classes or fitness videos, or you can just put on your shoes and hit the pavement.

The Person This Diet Is Best For Anyone who hates to diet but doesn't mind getting her rear in gear and working out.

OPRAH'S BOOT CAMP

We think that Oprah must have been a Marine drill sergeant in her former life. No one else could expect us to go through such a grueling routine as Oprah's Boot Camp. In this program, Oprah started with Bob Greene's *Total Body Makeover* and kicked it up a notch—and we don't mean like Emeril does. Instead of seven workouts per week, we get eight. We are supposed to do aerobics once a day for four days, twice a day for two days, and rest on the seventh. If you think that's tough, wait until you see what you'll eat!

Oprah stresses the elimination of all the white stuff from our diets. That means no rice, no flour, and no sugar. Ouch! But if you can get past the pain principle, you'll realize that whole grains are healthier, and sugar never gave anyone smoother skin or a better sex life. You are permitted two fruits daily and all the green vegetables you want. You can eat lean proteins and include just a little bit of good fat daily.

For the first four weeks, this is all you'll eat. You don't even get whole grains—no oatmeal, whole-grain bread, not even a grain of brown rice. Assuming you make it through the first four weeks, you can gradually add the whole grains back into your diet.

Now, we know what you are thinking. At first glance, Oprah's Boot Camp sounds really difficult, and a whole lot like Dr. Atkins. And the first part of the diet doesn't seem balanced, so why would Oprah suggest that we do something so restrictive? We thought she loved us! Maybe it's tough love, because while the plan does start out difficult, it gets easier, and ultimately, it really works. If you can survive, you really will feel better, and you really will lose weight. One of our own members had this to say after she completed the twelve-week program:

> This plan would work great if we, like those featured on Oprah's show, had a boss who worked out with us and would get mad at us if we cheated (I mean who wants to make Oprah mad?), had gym equipment at work, and time set aside to exercise. And like Oprah, had people to prepare meals and personal trainers to come to our home and help us work out on the Cadillac of Pilates equipment. I know Oprah works hard and like everyone has to carve time into her day for stuff like that, but still . . .

Between us chicks, for us, Oprah's Boot Camp looked so difficult that we didn't even make the attempt. Unless we had Oprah herself cracking her whip behind us, we just knew there was no way we were going to be able to stick to it. As diets go, this one is a little too strict for our taste. What ever happened to just using a little common sense and eating normal foods in reasonable portions? We think that this diet might be successful for chicks who don't have a lot of weight to lose, because they won't have to stick to it long. But if you're aiming for a thirty-, fifty-, or hundred-pound loss, we don't see how anybody could stay in Oprah's Boot Camp that long! Here are some thoughts, questions, and concerns from our chicks in Boot Camp who survived to tell the tale.

Q: I know I can't live on green vegetables; they all taste the same to me. Can I at least add tomatoes? What about dairy, such as yogurt? Isn't calcium supposed to be good for weight loss?

3FC: Although the plan does say just green vegetables, we did notice that official Boot Camp members, including Oprah's own staffers, are eating other nonstarchy vegetables. You can have tomatoes, bell peppers, summer squash, eggplant, and more. Once you increase your list of veggies, you can create a lot of really good meals. Most people are also eating some dairy, though they limit it to low-fat or nonfat types, and usually have no more than one cup daily. This seems to work better for the group. And you are right; studies have shown that the calcium in dairy products can help weight loss. However, it needs to be in a dairy product; the effect has not been the same with calcium supplements. We think you should grab your yogurt and not worry about it.

Q: How do I know which to choose? **Make the Connection, Total Body Makeover,** *or Oprah's Boot Camp?*

3FC: Begin by asking yourself what your goals are and how much effort you want to put into this process. If you want quick results and are willing to severely limit your food choices, Oprah's Boot Camp is the way to go. It's tough to follow, but you will see results. If you can't handle the limited food choices but are willing to work out, go for *Total Body Makeover.* You'll work hard, but you can eat what you want to eat, within reason, of course. A lot of women prefer a balanced diet, with a gentle push and easy-to-follow guidelines. *Make the Connection* is a great place to start, and it's a classic!

oprah's boot camp in an eggshell

Professional Counseling None.

Support System Message board on Oprah's Web site at www .oprah.com and the option of creating buddy groups on her Web site. No official interaction or guidance.

Fitness Factor *Lots!* Intensive workout, no slacking.

Family-Friendly Not very. Oprah's diet plan is very strict and, with its lack of grains and its other restrictions, particularly in the first four weeks, not balanced for the whole family. Be prepared to feed your family extra foods.

Pros If you can stick it out, it really works.

Cons It is rather extreme at first and may be difficult to stick to.

$$ Cheap! You should buy Bob's *Total Body Makeover* book, dumbbells, and ordinary healthy foods.

The Person This Diet Is Best For Someone who is seriously dedicated, understands the commitment, and is looking for quick initial results.

DR. PHIL'S ULTIMATE WEIGHT-LOSS SOLUTION

Have you ever given up on a diet because the weight loss was too slow? If you're anything like us, the answer to that question is probably *Duh! Of course!* We've all been hung up with instant gratification blues at some point in our lives. Dieting isn't usually a whole lot of fun, doesn't taste rich, sweet, or creamy, and generally doesn't give us overnight results. Going in, we know that, and we think we're prepared to stick with it, for better or worse, until fat do we part. As soon as the scale gives us a disappointing performance two weeks in a row, we're packing our bags and moving on to another diet that works better. It's not the diet that failed us, though; it's our unrealistic expectations.

Lucky for us, Oprah has delivered straight-talking Dr. Phil to set us back on the straight and narrow path to long-term success! Dr. Phil has heard every excuse, bad habit, and dirty diet secret in the fat chick arsenal, and he exposes them all in his book *The Ultimate Weight Solution.*

Diet and exercise are the bottom line of weight loss, but emotional, psychological, and philosophical hang-ups are the real obstacles that can stop us cold. Dr. Phil's book helps prepare us for the reality of the dieting experience. He strips away the fantasies and expectations and excuses and forces us to look the idea of long-term weight loss right in the face from the beginning, so that disappointment won't knock us off course later.

The information that Dr. Phil gives us is the same common sense that we all have but sometimes don't pay attention to because we can't always manage to see the forest for the treats! The sad fact is, as pointed out in his book, statistics show that diet programs have only a 5 percent success rate. Dr. Phil, however, claims an 80 percent success rate with his patients. What is his secret to success? In a word, self-control.

The predominant themes in Dr. Phil's Seven Keys to Weight Loss Freedom are all based on self-control and basic diet and exercise common sense. It sounds simple because it is. But if losing weight is this easy, why aren't we all at goal weight? Well, Dr. Phil says because the truth hurts! Dr. Phil reaffirms what we all know but are in denial about. This isn't going to be quick and easy, so put those flashy headlines out of your head. This book delivers the raw facts.

Dr. Phil teaches us realistic expectations. A healthy body is realistic, and a perfect body isn't. Realistic goals are a must. If you're five feet tall, don't reach for a six-foot model's physique. There is no diet that will turn Danny DeVito into Brad Pitt. We also shouldn't expect to lose five pounds a week. It's sad but true that we're inundated with hype about fast "fat" loss that is no more than water weight fluctuation.

So the good news is that you will reach your goals through Dr. Phil's Seven Keys to Weight Loss Freedom. As you learn the keys, you will become more focused and in control of your weight loss. The keys will teach you how to think proactively, gain control of emotional eating, prepare your environment, and eliminate its triggers, overcome impulse eating, make the best food choices, exercise effectively and *like* it, and develop a support network. Whew! We get exhausted just thinking about it, which is to say, this book isn't exactly light reading.

Of these seven keys, five of them involve personal steps that you will work toward on your own. The other two keys are the diet and exercise program, which we'll take a peek at now.

Dr. Phil's eating plan is called High-Response Cost, High-Yield Nutrition. It is compiled of foods that will help you lose weight and gain control of your eating habits. Dr. Phil points out that most diets today either cut out food groups entirely, or concoct special combinations of foods to bring about rapid water weight loss. While these diets work in the short term, they don't allow you to go back to your old eating habits without gaining the weight back. Dr. Phil's approach teaches you how to control your eating patterns instead. All foods are either "high-response cost, high-yield" or "low-response cost, low-yield." These aren't exactly catchy phrases, but once you understand the definitions, you can call them whatever you like!

The high-response cost, high-yield foods are, in general, foods that either take some time to eat or digest, or take awhile to prepare. They are also nutritious, such as the Shrimp Zucchini Salad on page 219. These are foods that you won't grab on the go and scarf down without thinking about it. Vegetables, fruits, meats, and whole grains are good examples. Low-response cost, low-yield foods are the processed, convenient foods that don't require much cooking or effort to prepare or digest. These are generally empty calories, or otherwise nonnutritious foods, such as candy bars, cheeseburgers, chips, etc. You can choke down these foods on impulse, and they can be in your belly before your tongue ever knows what hit it. You need to avoid these foods as much as possible.

The daily portions are mapped out for all food groups, such as three servings of protein, two servings of dairy, and four servings of vegetables. No groups are left out. If it's too difficult to keep up with the exact requirements, you can divide your plate into four equal sections. One fourth of your plate gets a protein, one fourth gets a starch, and the remaining half gets fruits or vegetables. You still need to learn portion control, though. No volcano stacks of rice on a fourth of an industrial-sized dinner platter!

Intentional exercise is another crucial key of Dr. Phil's weight-loss plan. We've heard it over and over, but here it is again. Exercise is a priority for anybody who wants to lose weight and successfully keep it off! As Dr. Phil so delicately puts it, "You must stop living like a lazy slug." The ratio of activity to eating has to be level in order to keep the weight off. The more you exercise, the stronger you will get, and the more control you will have over your body. Dr. Phil also contends that exercise will help reduce our urges to overeat.

Dr. Phil also tells us very clearly that we should make sure we get at least three to four hours a week of moderate exercise, which is pleasure walking, housecleaning, yard work, etc., and at least two to three hours of vigorous exercise per week. Vigorous exercise is aerobics, swimming, weight lifting, strenuous sports, etc. A lot of people don't want to hear that, but we can always count on Dr. Phil to give it to us straight!

Now, we know that Dr. Phil can rub some chicks the wrong way. And it's true, he is a little bit of a know-it-all, and he can sometimes make us feel like we're listening to a lecture from Dad. But regardless of what anybody thinks about Dr. Phil's personality, he really does have a lot going for him in the world of weight-loss motivation. Dr. Phil has his feet on the ground psychologically, and he's not afraid to tell us everything that we need to know but don't want to hear. He really will help you "get real" about weight loss and realistic expectations and goals. His program is helpful for anybody who has dieted and failed in the past, which is, like, 105 percent of us.

Lastly, his words stick. Compare with an infomercial: thirty minutes of inspirational talk and I'm ready to become a real estate magnate and live in Hawaii. The next morning, I've already lost the phone number. Dr. Phil digs in deeper and helps you approach weight loss logically. Here's some of what our Dr. Phil chicks had to say, when we asked them to get real about getting real.

Q: It sounds like Dr. Phil thinks that everybody has a problem with compulsive or emotional overeating. I don't have a problem with food, so can't I just follow the diet and skip the tongue-lashing?

3FC: If you can go straight through the diet without any issues, yeah, sure! Chances are, though, we all have *some* sort of issue or we wouldn't be overweight in the first place. The basic weight-loss plan can stand alone from the rest of the system, just as the keys to mental and emotional success can be worked with another diet and exercise plan. However, they truly are meant to work together. If you are only interested in the diet and exercise plan, do yourself a favor and spend a couple of extra hours reading *all* the keys, whether or not you take the quizzes, as they could mean a big payoff on your bottom line, no pun intended!

If you really don't want to work through all the keys, then don't. But if you have problems sticking to plan, or if you develop negative feelings while on this plan, you need to give in and review the keys. Unlike your bathroom scale, the Seven Keys to Weight Loss Freedom are very forgiving and you can always go back for a second helping.

Q: Are meal-replacement drinks okay? Dr. Phil considers them low-response because they are a convenience food, right?

3FC: A meal-replacement drink would fit the definition of low-response since you only have to pop the lid and kick it back. However, if it is a nutritious meal-replacement drink, then Dr. Phil says it is okay in moderation.

Moderation does not mean a drink for breakfast, a drink for lunch, and a sensible dinner. Drinks and bars are both okay if you're in a pinch and have no other choice. Look at it this way: if you are in a situation where you would normally grab fast food or a low-response, low-yield snack, go for the meal-replacement drink. Check your labels and make sure the calories are not too high, that you are getting a fair amount of protein and fiber, and that there is not an abundance of sugar.

Q: The diet allows one tablespoon of fat per day? How can I manage that? Get real, Dr. Phil!

3FC: That requirement is for added fat, like olive oil or nuts. You'll already have some fat in meats, eggs, fish, and low-fat dairy products, so you will have additional fat in the diet. Your extra fat for cooking or garnishing will be cut down.

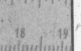

dr. phil–approved low-fat lovelies

1. Grill or broil meat whenever you can to reduce the fat.
2. Poach or steam meat or vegetables in a broth.
3. Make a light cheese sauce with low-fat cheese and skim milk, with a pinch of flour.
4. Use fat-free marinades or high-flavor vinegars on meats and veggies, and sauté with nonfat cooking spray.
5. In the skillet, try using a teaspoon of olive oil per serving, and add fruit juice or a splash of wine to aid in flavor and moisture.
6. Top foods with salsa instead of higher-fat choices, like butter and cheeses.
7. Use a spritz of butter spray, or butter sprinkles on your plate.
8. Use a steamer for fish and vegetables.
9. Try mustards and fat-free dressings instead of mayonnaise.

dr. phil in an eggshell

Professional Counseling None face-to-face, but you have the complete, in-depth program from the doctor himself.

Support System Dr. Phil has his own on-line community on his Web site at www.drphil.com, plus he outlines the importance of a support system in one of his seven keys.

Fitness Factor Intentional exercise is one of the seven keys and vital to the success of the program.

Family-Friendly Absolutely. There is nothing on this plan that you and your family cannot do for the rest of your natural life.

Pros This is a regular way of eating, so it will not require switching plans when you get to maintenance. There are no food groups dropped from the plan.

Cons The diet plan is based on foods that take longer to prepare. Cooking isn't always easy with a busy lifestyle. Convenience foods are to be avoided. The plan is heavy on the psychological aspect of weight loss, so it takes a while to absorb.

$$ While whole foods can be more expensive, this program poo-poos convenience and junk foods, which tend to be expensive, so you will probably save money.

The Person This Diet Is Best For Someone who has problems with emotional eating or who has a strong history of diet failure and is patient enough to take a long look at herself. Also good for people who like to cook.

recipes from the front lines

BOB GREENE MAKES
THE CONNECTION

Breakfast doesn't have to be tedious, involve anything with "Grand Slam" in the title, or stick to your ribs all morning. Try something new that is quick and light.

tomato basil eggs

Serves 1

1 small slice tomato, or 1 sliced cherry tomato
1 fresh basil leaf, chopped
1 egg
Dash salt and black pepper to taste
¼ ounce Neufchâtel cheese (light cream cheese) cut into two
    cubes, ½ inch each

Preheat oven to 425°F. Spray a ramekin with cooking spray. Lay tomato slice in bottom of ramekin, and top with chopped basil. In a small bowl, lightly beat egg with salt and pepper. Pour egg over tomato and basil. Gently lay Neufchâtel cubes on top of egg. Bake in the oven for about 10 minutes, or until puffed and very lightly browned.

Per serving: 97 calories, 7 grams fat, 2 grams carbs, 0 fiber, 7 grams protein

DR. PHIL'S ULTIMATE WEIGHT-LOSS SOLUTION

Here's a recipe that is full of flavor and easy to make, and still fits the bill of high-response, high-yield fare. This salad is simple but packs a lot of flavor.

shrimp zucchini salad

Serves 1

½ teaspoon minced garlic
2 teaspoons red bell pepper, finely minced
½ teaspoon lemon zest
2 tablespoons vegetable broth
4 ounces shrimp, peeled and deveined
1 tablespoon fresh lemon juice
1½ teaspoons canola oil
Dash salt
Dash black pepper
1 small baby zucchini, about 3 ounces, thinly sliced
1 cup mixed salad greens
½ ounce freshly shaved Parmesan cheese

Sauté garlic, red bell pepper, and lemon zest in vegetable broth for about 30 seconds. Add shrimp and continue to sauté until shrimp is done. If necessary, add another tablespoon of broth. Remove to small dish and set aside.

Combine lemon juice, canola oil, salt, and pepper in a small mixing bowl. Add sliced zucchini and toss well to coat. Place salad greens on a salad plate or bowl. Top with the zucchini

• *Continued on next page* •

mixture and shrimp, and toss lightly. Sprinkle with shaved Parmesan cheese. Make sure you use a good quality cheese, for best flavor.

Per serving: 297 calories, 14 grams fat, 12 carbs, 3 grams fiber, 31 grams protein

Words to Live By

My idea of heaven is a great big baked potato and someone to share it with. —OPRAH WINFREY

We can't become what we need to be by remaining what we are.
—OPRAH WINFREY

mediterranean chicks don't get fat
the mediterranean diet

DESPITE OUR NATIONAL obsession with dieting, Americans are just getting fatter. In fact, Americans have the highest obesity rate in the world. France, on the other hand, has one of the lowest. The French people, along with others from Mediterranean countries, are thinner than us, even though they eat foods that we would consider taboo on many diets, such as croissants stuffed with Brie cheese, chocolate after every meal, or baklava for dessert. How do they eat all that good food and still stay thin?

This hot topic has been the subject of several recent books, the most notable being *French Women Don't Get Fat* by Mireille Guiliano. In her book, Guiliano describes the typical French lifestyle and the way the French manage food and daily activities to maintain their Parisian model physiques. Dr. Will Clower is the author of *The Fat Fallacy*, a guide to eating and living the French way to attain weight loss and better health. Here are the main principles of this eating philosophy that will help us stay Paris thin, even though we're eating dinner in Des Moines.

- **Breakfast.** Start your day off with a memorable breakfast. Take your time and enjoy it, and your breakfast experience will improve the rest of your day physically, psychologically, and emotionally.

- **Portion control.** Mediterraneans do not overload their plates with pasta, eat footlong overstuffed subs, or devour Grand Slam breakfasts. Their croissants are half the size of ours. An after-dinner chocolate is just one small, sinfully rich square.

- **Eat slowly.** Many people on the other side of the globe take the time to savor their foods; they turn their meals into memorable experiences. They don't gulp down their dinner so fast that they can't remember what they ate. By eating slowly, and consuming moderate amounts of fat, they give their bodies a chance to become full and satisfied on smaller portions.

- **Eat fresh foods.** Highly processed foods are not as popular in other countries as they are in America. Instead, fresh markets, filled with fruits and vegetables, are preferred over cans and boxes in supermarkets. If you do eat packaged foods, read the ingredient labels to make sure there's natural food inside, not a lot of chemicals. Dr. Clower says, "If it ain't food, don't eat it." This goes for artificial sweeteners, food colors, and any other additives.

- **Attitude.** In Mediterranean countries, mealtime is an experience to be appreciated. In America, our meals are typically treated as a necessity, with little thought given to the sensual properties of the food or the social joys of the company. Love your food at mealtimes, and the food will love you back!

- **Exercise.** It's impossible to get away from this requirement, no matter where you live. The French, and other Europeans, tend to walk much more than we do. They are constantly on the go, where we are usually stuck in traffic. Make a conscious effort to move more.

The "Mediterranean diet" is a regionally inspired plan that is more a style of eating than a structured diet. This diet can be confusing because it isn't all laid out with serving sizes or points, which we've become accustomed to when choosing diets. You're pretty much on your own when choosing foods and portions on the Mediterranean diet, but it's not really as scary as it sounds, and the food selections make it worth the extra effort to exercise moderation. If you spend a few weeks on the Mediterranean, you'll probably never want to go home again!

While the Mediterranean diet is not specifically a weight-loss plan, like Weight Watchers, you can easily lose weight on it. You'll eat a lot of fresh fruits, vegetables, and grains. You won't eat much meat or many processed foods. Some of us chicks are skeptical about eating anything that doesn't get served up with a basket of fries. Don't be afraid; it's not all hummus and eggplant. You're going to be able to eat pasta and even pizza, but don't expect to eat like you do at your local pizzeria. This diet takes its inspiration from the old, traditional Mediterranean foods, which do not include cheesy bread or hot wings.

Obviously, the Mediterranean diet is based on the foods of the countries that border the Mediterranean Sea, including Spain, France, Turkey, Greece, Italy, Egypt, Morocco, and others. There isn't just one diet that all of these countries follow, but they all do share some common characteristics. Each of these shared components should be included, because they all work together to provide maximum health benefits. Studies have shown that adopting just one or two of these characteristics did not always make a weight-loss difference, but including most or all of the changes did.

PRINCIPLES OF THE MEDITERRANEAN DIET

- This is mostly a plant-based diet. You will eat lots of fruits, vegetables, whole grains, and legumes.

- Fish and other seafood may be eaten a few times per week. Chicken is eaten less often, and beef and other meats are limited to just once a month. The preferred source of protein is legumes.
- Fruit is the preferred dessert and is usually eaten plain or just lightly sweetened. Lightly sweetened doesn't mean floating in a cobbler. You may have traditional sweets once or twice a week, so you are not completely giving up your treats.
- Chicks get to drink one glass of red wine every day. Men can have two glasses. A glass a day does not equal a bottle on the weekend. Moderation!
- You can have dairy every day, though it should be consumed in moderation to reduce the amounts of saturated fat in your diet. Think yogurt and cheese rather than milk.
- This is not a low-fat diet but allows moderate levels of mainly monounsaturated fats such as olive oil and nut oils. Saturated fats are very limited, and trans fats should always be avoided.
- The foods you will eat are generally fresh, whole, natural, and not heavily processed. You won't eat a lot of faux foods or high-sodium frozen dinners and condiments. Good-bye, Oscar Mayer. Hello, Jolly Green Giant.
- Regular exercise is just as important as the various food suggestions.

The White Stuff

It's hard to escape the warnings of the evils of the "white stuff"—warnings that have been dished out by everyone from Atkins to Oprah. White stuff includes refined flour products such as bread and pasta, as well as sugar and white rice. Whole-wheat products are definitely higher in nutrition and should be included whenever possible, especially since many Americans don't usually get whole grains from any other source. Yet when we think of real Italian pasta, we don't envision the brown pasta that graces our own supermarket shelves. In fact, the bulk of all pasta eaten in Mediterranean countries is white and has been for two thousand years. At one point, whole-wheat products were considered the food of the pauper, while white wheat was the food of the prince. Even couscous, a staple of countries including Morocco and Israel, is just a semolina pasta product. So Mediterranean people have managed to retain their good health while eating the white stuff. Even sugary sweets can be consumed once or twice a week, or on special occasions. Who couldn't resist the occasional serving of baklava? It's the next best thing to pecan pie! The lesson learned? Choose whole wheat when possible, limit portion sizes, but don't be too afraid of the white stuff.

mediterranean comforts

One of the first hurdles of the Mediterranean diet is accepting the fact that we have to give up our traditional ideas about what comfort food is, down here in the Bible Belt. So for all of us who don't feel loving until there are cookies in the oven, here's a list of Mediterranean substitutions for the comforts of home.

The Mediterranean Diet	Versus	The Bible Belt Diet
pita bread		buttermilk biscuits
olive oil		Crisco
eggplant, roasted		baby back ribs
over a fire pit		catfish and hush puppies
shrimp scampi		Tater Tots
couscous		chicken nuggets
roasted chicken		corn dog
shish kebab		

Since this diet contains very few processed foods, which are usually calorie- and/or fat-laden, you will probably eat fewer calories overall, while eating higher quantities of food that keep you satisfied. Recent studies have shown that the moderate-fat Mediterranean diet is more successful than a standard low-fat diet for losing weight and keeping it off. Many believe that this is because the diet is easier to stick to long-term because the food is so good. What other diet encourages eating pizza, Greek salads, and honey-soaked figs? Chances are you probably won't need to count calories when you adopt this style of eating, since nearly everything you eat will be good for you and fairly low in calories. As always, you just need to watch your portion sizes. It would be difficult to apply the Mediterranean diet to low-carb plans such as Atkins, because those plans are too restrictive and would not allow all of the components of the Mediterranean diet. However, you can apply the characteristics of the Mediterranean diet to many other diet plans, such as Weight Watchers or the South Beach diet.

Are you still confused? Or are you salivating and wondering how you can apply this philosophy to your own diet plan? If you want to know more, here are some well-tanned Mediterranean chicks to tell us how this diet helped them lose weight.

meet the mediterranean chicks

Shannon from Georgia

Our family's tight budget has often meant spaghetti dinners made from jarred spaghetti sauce and a huge platter of pasta. It was cheap, filling, and easy to overeat. Before I knew it, I weighed 236 pounds. When I heard about the Mediterranean diet, I thought that I'd be able to find a way to continue our spaghetti dinners but still lose weight. I don't know what I was expecting, maybe a fat-burning herb seasoning. I started experimenting with recipes that I found on-line and was thrilled that they fit into our budget. I had to work to curb my pasta habit, but I learned more about portion control than I ever knew before. I've been eating more vegetables and less pasta, and have lost 60 pounds so far.

Karen from Tennessee

I discovered the Mediterranean diet by accident. My husband is Greek, and I was researching Greek cuisine so that I could cook some of his favorite childhood dishes, instead of our usual fish and chips or meatloaf and mashed potato dinners. We started eating more shellfish, grains, and vegetables such as eggplant. I really loved the food and it was fun to surprise my husband with what I was learning. He was first to notice that I was losing a little weight, and we knew it had to be the new food. I thought, "Hey, there must be something to this!" and after Googling Greek diets, I learned about the Mediterranean diet and how popular it was. I kept on cooking, and started exercising more, and went down three dress sizes!

Diane from Oregon

I'm a vegetarian, so it's been kind of hard to find a good diet plan that I could live with. Most of the diets are geared toward meat eaters. My doctor recommended the Mediterranean diet and said he'd been following it for years. I thought it was confusing at first, but after I got the hang of it, I liked it and saw results quickly. The foods were things I've eaten for years, but the guidelines put the plan into perspective for me, so I ended up eating less and making better choices. My doctor was so thrilled with my results that he put my picture on the bulletin board in his office to show other patients!

Q: I'm very happy counting points because it is the easiest way for me to lose weight. Can I do the Mediterranean diet while on Weight Watchers? There seems to be a lot of olive oil on this plan.

3FC: The Weight Watchers Flex plan is so flexible that it's easy to apply the Mediterranean concept to it. You just need to count the point values of the foods you choose. There is one stumbling block to watch out for. Weight Watchers members frequently substitute highly processed, nonfat foods to conserve points, such as fat-free sour cream or other dairy products. Frozen diet meals, such as Weight Watchers Smart Ones dinners, are also a popular choice of Weight Watchers members. Unfortunately, these products are so highly processed that they should be avoided on the Mediterranean diet. You'll want to eat freshly prepared meals using natural ingredients, such as the polenta recipe on page 234.

The Weight Watchers Core plan may seem ideal for the Mediterranean diet, until you consider what you have to avoid. The Core plan requires a lot of vegetables, whole grains, and lean meats, but it also prohibits many fruits, all sugars, red wine, and some of the carbs that the Mediterranean diet needs to be balanced. Plus, it encourages only fat-free dairy, such as nonfat cheeses and sour cream. You can't get all of the components of the Mediterranean diet into the Core plan.

Q: How do I do Phase 1 of the South Beach diet if I'm eating the Mediterranean diet with it? There are too many grains. Can I skip them?

3FC: Phases 2 and 3 of the South Beach diet are very similar to the Mediterranean diet, but Phase 1 is a challenge. On the Mediterranean diet you will eat lots of fresh fruit, whole grains, and a glass of wine each day, which we know are taboo on Phase 1 of South Beach. You can do Phase 1 as it is in the book, and then make the transition to Phase 2 by choosing Med-diet-friendly foods. The purpose of Phase 1 is to help kill your carb cravings and to get rid of a few pounds of water weight. If you don't need this assistance, more power to you! Just move directly to Phase 2.

There are a few things to keep in mind when blending the Mediterranean with South Beach. You may need to curb your string cheese or ricotta crème habit. The Med diet doesn't allow quite as much dairy as is allowed on South Beach. Another obstacle is the South Beach diet frozen dinners and sandwich wraps that have become popular. One glance at the half-page-long ingredient labels on these products is all it takes to realize that they are not the natural, unprocessed foods that you should be eating with your new lifestyle. However, you can eat very satisfying meals of grilled fish, lentil chili (page 235), pasta with tomato and vegetable sauce, and fresh fruits.

a typical south beach diet phase 2 day with mediterranean flair

Breakfast ¾ cup blueberries with ½ cup nonfat, sugar-free vanilla yogurt, sprinkled with a tablespoon of wheat germ

Lunch Roasted tomato soup, salad, and a bowl of fresh grapes for dessert

Snack Hummus and pita wedges

Dinner Spicy Lentil Chili, whole-wheat pita wedges for dipping; fruit salad for dessert; a glass of red wine with or after dinner

---

Q: I love Mexican food, but Mexico isn't exactly a Mediterranean country. Can I eat enchiladas and my other favorite spicy foods on this plan?

3FC: Absolutely! Many Mexican dishes rely on tomatoes, peppers, onions, black beans, and other vegetables. You'll probably want to choose vegetarian options most of the time and limit dishes with a lot of beef and saturated fats in them. But be realistic: you probably won't find many suitable choices at your local taco shack. Look for restaurants that offer authentic Mexican cuisine, and ask questions if you are not sure what's in the dishes. Remember the basic guidelines:

fresh food, portion control, and taking your time to enjoy. Many Mexican-style foods are already designed as individual portions, such as enchiladas or fajitas. Add a homemade salsa for flavor and freshness. You might even want to explore Spanish foods, such as paella. If you like spicy foods, you can zing up just about any Mediterranean dish with hot spices, such as our hummus recipe on page 236.

Q: I've been on the Web doing searches for Mediterranean diet and I can't find anything about weight loss. I've been on South Beach, but I miss my carbs. Can I really expect to lose weight if I eat this way?

3FC: The Mediterranean diet can be used for weight loss, or it can just be a lifestyle choice. We like that there are no forbidden foods except junk foods on a diet plan like this. You can have a mixture of whole and refined grains. You can eat fruits, potatoes, and other foods that some other diet plans don't permit. The key is portion control. The people who live in Mediterranean regions are much healthier because they eat more natural foods and fewer processed foods that contain chemicals and mystery products. They use good fats such as olive oil. They also practice portion control as a matter of course. Americans, in general, just eat too much! That is what we have to learn to get away from. For many people, weight is less about what we eat than how much we eat.

Most of the Web sites devoted to the Med diet focus on it not as a way to lose weight but as a way to regain health, and especially to protect our hearts. It's a healthier way to live. However, there is a book called *The Mediterranean Diet: Newly Revised and Updated* by Marissa Cloutier and Eve Adamson that does emphasize weight loss. It discusses various foods you should look for and even includes a few sample menus and recipes. Most of the books on the Mediterranean diet do not offer menus, so you need to base your choices around your own needs.

If you want to lose weight, decide how many calories you want to consume, then plan your Mediterranean menu to stay within your target count. It's the calories that count for weight loss in the end. And, as always, exercise is very important for weight loss. You are in complete control and can choose the foods you enjoy. It takes a little planning, but you learn more that way.

Q: I don't like wine and don't understand why it's required by this diet plan. Shouldn't we avoid alcohol when dieting?

3FC: Red wine is loaded with antioxidants and has been shown to help reduce the risk of heart disease when it is consumed regularly and in moderation. It is common to have a glass of red wine with dinner in Mediterranean countries. Do you have to drink it? No, it's not required, it's a personal choice. Plus it won't help you lose weight any faster. A lot of people don't like to drink alcohol, or they just don't like the flavor of wine. Purple grape juice also contains antioxidants, but you would have to drink more of it to get the same benefit, which would add up to more calories. Pomegranate juice may have even more antioxidants than red wine, and it tastes good!

Q: Since there isn't a menu or plan with this diet, how do I know how much to eat?

3FC: Now is a good time to learn what food portions should be. We've become so used to platters of pasta as served in restaurants that we don't know when to stop eating at home. Don't be afraid to use measuring cups until you familiarize yourself with correct portions. Then you can eyeball it. You don't need to count calories or carbs when you choose to eat like the French or other Mediterraneans, but you do need to get control of the amount of food you eat. Train yourself to eat until you are just satisfied and never stuffed. Don't take seconds, even if your grandma insists. Limit yourself to small amounts of rich foods, such as cream sauces or breads. If you are still hungry, help yourself to more vegetables, or have a fruit for dessert. It shouldn't take long before this way of eating comes naturally to you.

size matters

The French are known for love, romance, thin women, and rich foods, and they do it so well. They know something important that we Americans try to deny: size matters. Smaller really is better! Try our tips for portion control, so you too can savor the finer things in life, a little at a time.

- Fresh fruit is often portion-controlled by Mother Nature. Enjoy a fresh whole banana, apple, peach, or other fruit, instead of fruit salad, applesauce, or other processed fruit that arrives in a large tub.
- Put your large dinner plates in storage, and use the salad or luncheon plates instead. Since we tend to portion out foods by how much will fit on our plates, we usually eat less if using a smaller plate.
- Put a little less food on your plate than you think you will eat. Lay your fork down between bites, and chew slowly. You probably won't need to get another portion. If you do, make sure it's a healthy choice.
- When dining out, choose an appetizer as your main dish, or a child-sized entrée. You may even split a regular entrée with your companion. Just don't order a full-sized entrée for yourself if you think you may eat it all.

mediterranean diet in an eggshell

Professional Counseling None. You'll rely on your own sensibilities to get you through.

Support System Not really. You may find a few forums on-line that offer support for the Mediterranean diet, including 3FC. But there isn't anything official out there.

Fitness Factor Exercise is a main component of the Mediterranean diet, though you are on your own in making fitness choices.

Family-Friendly Very, since it is healthy and delicious for every member of the family.

$$ Very affordable because you'll eat little meat but a lot of vegetables and grains. You can also eat plenty of lentils and other legumes that can be purchased cheaply in bulk.

Pros Easier to stick to than most diets because the food is so good, and you can easily maintain it for life.

Cons You'll probably spend more time food shopping and in the kitchen since you will be preparing fresher foods from scratch, instead of depending on a lot of convenience foods.

The Person This Diet Is Best For Someone concerned about overall health and especially heart disease and cancer. Perfect for foodies who love this type of cuisine.

recipes from the front lines

This salad is low in Weight Watchers points but high in flavor. It is a perfect way to incorporate some of the Mediterranean diet into your Weight Watchers plan.

red pepper and goat cheese salad with polenta medallions

Serves 3

1 roasted red bell pepper, from a jar, cut in long strips
1 small tomato, chopped
½ cup fresh basil leaves, torn
½ small onion, sliced thin
2 tablespoons balsamic vinegar
1 tablespoon olive oil
Salt and pepper to taste
1 head bibb lettuce, or 1 bag of salad mix
1 ounce goat cheese
6 slices (¼-inch thick) purchased sun-dried tomato polenta

Combine red pepper strips, tomato, basil, onion, balsamic vinegar, and olive oil in a medium bowl. Add salt and pepper to taste. Cover and let sit at room temperature for about an hour. Or prepare in advance and chill until serving time. The tomatoes will release juices as they marinate, to create more liquid for the dressing.

Prepare polenta: Spray a nonstick skillet with cooking spray and heat over medium high heat. Add the polenta slices and carefully cook until lightly golden on each side.

To serve: Divide lettuce among 3 large plates. Top with pepper mixture. Sprinkle with goat cheese. Place polenta slices on the side of the plates and serve.

Per serving: 118 calories, 8 grams fat, 7 grams protein, 23 carbohydrates, 4 WW points

Enjoy the best of both worlds with this South Beach-Mediterranean blend. It's got everything you need—taste *and* nutrition—to help you lose weight and feel satisfied. This meal is so good, you won't remember that you're dieting.

spicy lentil chili

Serves 6

1 cup red lentils
Water
2 tablespoons olive oil
½ cup onion, diced
¼ cup celery, finely chopped
2 tablespoons garlic, chopped
1 medium tomato, cored and diced
2 cups canned vegetable broth
1 tablespoon Tabasco sauce
⅛ teaspoon turmeric
⅛ teaspoon cumin

● *Continued on next page* ●

⅛ teaspoon cayenne pepper
1 teaspoon sea salt
½ teaspoon black pepper
⅛ teaspoon chili powder

Bring lentils and 2 cups of water to a boil over high heat. Remove from heat. Place half the lentils and water in a blender or food processor and puree. Set aside.

Heat olive oil in a stockpot or Dutch oven over medium heat. Add onions and stir until they begin to soften. Add celery and garlic and continue to stir and cook for about 5 minutes. Add chopped tomatoes and cook an additional 5 minutes. Add vegetable broth, Tabasco sauce, and seasonings. Continue to heat until mixture begins to simmer. Stir in pureed lentils and reserved whole lentils and water mixture. Stir well and cook until lentils are tender, about 15 minutes. If chili is too thick, add additional water to thin.

Per serving: 226 calories, 6 grams fat, 12 grams protein, 34 grams carbs

---

Does the idea of hummus make you say *hmmmm*? Try our zesty recipe for a delicious and healthy hummus for snacks or entertaining. It also packs easily for a quick and healthy lunch at the office. Don't forget to pack the breath mints!

zesty red pepper hummus

Makes about 2 cups

1 can (16 ounces) chickpeas, drained and rinsed
2 cloves garlic, peeled and coarsely chopped
¼ cup tahini

½ cup roasted red bell peppers
2 tablespoons fresh lemon juice
1 tablespoon olive oil
½ teaspoon cayenne pepper, or to taste

Combine all ingredients in the bowl of a food processor and pulse until mixture is smooth. Add a little water, if necessary, to thin the mixture to the right consistency. Transfer to a serving bowl and serve at room temperature with raw vegetables or pita chips.

Per ¼-cup serving: 127 calories, 6 grams fat, 4 grams protein, 15 grams carbs

Words to Live By

Everything you see I owe to spaghetti. —SOPHIA LOREN

If I want a bite of chocolate cake, I will have it. I just won't eat the whole cake like I used to. —JUDITH LIGHT

radical chicks
weight-loss surgery

LISTEN, BEFORE WE BEGIN to talk about an approach to weight loss as radical as surgery, we want to make sure that everybody understands surgery is *not* a quick fix. It's not as easy as it looks on some reality TV shows, where you go under the knife, spend a few days in funny-looking bandages, recover in no time thanks to the magic of time-lapse filming, and then emerge gorgeous and thin, looking trim and slim in a little black dress and perfect hair while everyone stands around and applauds your remarkable transformation. This is the real world, not TV, and when it comes to radical procedures like weight-loss surgery, you need to understand the difference.

Every chick needs to sit down and do a lot of soul-searching before considering a surgical procedure. And it's important when you're weighing your pros and cons to understand that this is not a simple, painless alternative to the struggle of saying no to cream pies and super-size. In fact, the decision to have weight-loss surgery runs far deeper than wondering if you can still eat your burgers deluxe.

Weight-loss surgery (WLS) changes you not only physically but emotionally and socially as well, and once you make the decision to pursue this course, you can never take a day off. Failure to stick to the diet plan that accompanies weight-loss surgery doesn't just result in a sugar and guilt hangover; it can result in severe illness or even death.

So why do some chicks choose weight-loss surgery? Well, because they have nowhere else to turn. These procedures are intended for heavy hens who have tried every other weight-loss option and failed. WLS is their last resort to lose weight and regain their lives, and for many, that last chance pays off.

Amy, of 3FC, had weight-loss surgery in 2003. She reached the point where she felt WLS was her last chance. She had dieted for many years, sometimes successfully, but was never able to keep it off. She would resume her old eating habits, usually because of stress, and always regained the weight. We watched her struggle not only with her weight but with the emotional pain she felt because she was not able to get it under control. We had mixed feelings about WLS and felt it should be reserved for extreme cases, and had a difficult time accepting Amy's choice. We were scared she would not survive the surgery. We were confused that she could not just lose the weight by dieting, because she'd done it before. But eventually, we accepted the reality of her pain and realized that this was truly Amy's last chance, so we chose to support her, and while she did hit some significant stumbling blocks along the way, her surgery has worked out well for her in the long run.

While there are risks involved with weight-loss surgery, there are many benefits, and often the risks of remaining obese outweigh the potential danger of surgery. According to the American Obesity Association, there are more than thirty obesity-related illnesses that can damage the quality of life and even cause death. It is up to you and your doctor to decide if surgery is a good choice for you.

According to Mark Lockett, MD and assistant professor of surgery at East Tennessee State University, the benefits of weight-loss surgery can be substantial. "Candidates for weight-loss surgery are morbidly obese and most studies suggest their life expectancies are significantly shorter than similar patients who are not obese, on the range of ten years or so. If a patient makes it through the surgery and recovery period, and ninety-eight percent do, then their life expectancy should increase."

Once you and your doctor have decided on weight-loss surgery, you will have to decide which type of procedure works best for you. There are several available. There is no best method, although there is great debate on this point in the WLS world, and not all surgeons perform all methods. If you study your options and feel strongly about a method not offered by your surgeon, you should get a second opinion. This is a permanent change and a very personal decision and you need to be sure you are making the right choice so you have no regrets.

You can elect to have restrictive surgery, which limits the amount of food that can be eaten by removing or closing a portion of the stomach. You eat less and feel full quicker. With restrictive surgery, the only thing that changes is the size of the stomach pouch, and the outlet size, which delays the emptying of food into the larger portion of the stomach. Now, that gives new meaning to the idea of food that sticks to your ribs!

You might also consider a combination of restrictive and malabsorption surgery. This procedure restricts the size of the pouch, plus it reduces the amount of nutrients and calories that can be absorbed by the body. In this process, the intestines are rerouted to alter the digestive system. As a result, you can only eat the foods that count, like proteins and nutrient-rich carbohydrates. Junk food and sugar are out; protein shakes, lean meat, and green veggies are in. You will also have to take vitamins and calcium supplements for the rest of your life.

Two of the most popular weight-loss surgeries are adjustable gastric banding and the Roux-en-Y gastric bypass.

Adjustable gastric banding (AGB), commonly known as the Lap-Band, is accomplished with the surgical insertion of a hollow silicone band around the upper portion of the stomach. The band divides the stomach into two sections, divided by a small opening. The first and smaller portion of the stomach, above the band, holds what you eat. This is also the section of your stomach that has all the nerves that scream "Feed me!" to your brain. When it is full, your brain is satisfied and won't know or care that you had only a two-ounce protein shake for dinner. Food is slowly passed through the banded entrance into the lower, larger section of stomach. Here your food will be digested normally. The band can be loosened or tightened by removing or adding a saline solution. This type of surgery does not involve moving or removing any of your organs, and it can be reversed.

Roux-en-Y gastric bypass (RGB) is the most commonly performed gastric bypass surgery in the United States. It reduces your stomach size, limiting the amount of food you can eat at one time. In addition, part of your intestines will be bypassed during the digestive process, reducing the amount of calories and, unfortunately, nutrients that can be absorbed. This two-pronged approach is one of the most effective methods of weight-loss surgery, but it cannot be reversed.

These procedures have one thing in common; after surgery, you must eat only quality foods. Postsurgical nip and tuckers will eat a very low-calorie diet. Since you will be eating less, every bite counts. You will eat very little sugar or fat. Failure to restrict your diet can interfere with your weight loss or make you ill.

To be approved for surgery, you generally need to be about a hundred pounds overweight. Specifically, your BMI, or body mass index, should be forty or more. A lower BMI may be acceptable if you experience an obesity-related illness such as diabetes, heart disease, or sleep apnea. You also will have to pass a psychological exam and attend support group meetings before the surgery. You also should have exhausted all efforts at losing weight through calorie reduction and exercise on your own. Getting approved for surgery, including undergoing the exams, is a long process. Don't be surprised if you have to wait six to twelve months from your first visit until the procedure. So much for the quick-fix idea!

Even if you meet the weight requirements, weight-loss surgery may not be for you. Here are some of the top reasons why people are excluded as weight-loss surgery candidates:

- You're addicted to drugs or alcohol.
- You have not exhausted your weight-loss options with diet and exercise.
- You have a stomach disorder.
- You're not willing to stick to a strict postsurgery diet.

- You think losing weight will solve other problems in your life.
- You don't have a family that will support your lifestyle change.
- You aren't willing to attend postsurgical therapy and follow-up visits.
- You have an eating disorder.
- You're a junk food junkie and can't give it up. (Although one indulgence may make you so sick, that could change!)
- You think of weight-loss surgery as a cure and not a tool.

Surgery is and will remain a controversial method of weight loss. This is a personal decision, and you should spend a lot of time reviewing your options before you make it. And it's important to work with your surgeon. She has your best interests at heart, and she will be sharing this experience with you, so don't be afraid to ask her about your concerns.

We asked our radical chicks to share some of their personal highs and lows with weight-loss surgery.

meet the radical chicks

Amy 3FC from Tennessee

I had the Roux-en-Y weight-loss surgery in 2003. I'd reached a high of 285 pounds and was tired and frustrated with my inability to lose the weight. After careful consideration and discussions with my doctor, I decided to go with the surgery. Do I regret it? No, not anymore, but I do wish that I could have controlled my weight on my own.

I had a difficult time adjusting to the forced calorie control at first. Right after the surgery, I was convinced I'd made the wrong decision. I was depressed. I cried a lot, and I was angry with myself for going

• *Continued on next page* •

through with the surgery. I realized that I had been influenced by celebrity success stories. I thought that if the stars had done so well with surgery, so could I. Once it was done, though, reality set in and I realized that I hadn't been prepared at all for what I had done.

In the end, it all worked out. I had a tough time for the first nine months, but I adjusted and I'm now very happy that I had the surgery. I've lost more than 130 pounds, I'm no longer diabetic, my sleep apnea is gone, and I feel very little pain from my arthritis. I also recently sealed my success with a tummy tuck!

Dawna from California

I know that somewhere down the line there could be health ramifications we did not know about at the time I had my surgery, and I took that into account when making my decision. I know, however, that I would probably have been dead or certainly disabled and unable to work within a few years, had I not had the surgery. If and when untoward effects happen down the road, I will have had many more happy, healthy, productive years than I would have had without the surgery. It is a chance we all take.

Terri from Maine

Food no longer controls me, and it is a wonderful feeling! Also, after ten years of being infertile due to morbid obesity, I just gave birth to my baby girl in December!

Deborah from Oklahoma

My first surgery was a gastric stapling. The staples came out when they did an MRI on my back, so I was back to over three hundred pounds. Having gained all the weight back and having bad reflux problems from the first surgery's having been halfway removed, I had Roux-en-Y. I out-ate that one and gained all but forty pounds back. It still made me feel better healthwise, and I have learned that now I have to change what I do instead of trying to out-eat every effort. I don't regret it at all because I needed it at those times in my life. For many people it is such a life-changing experience, and it was for me also. I wasn't successful because I didn't follow the rules after my surgery. I drank regular pop, soups, anything that would go down easy and lots of it. Very stupid of me, but I did it, so now I'm losing weight again the low-cal method. Surgery is a great tool to help people get on track, but you have to take care.

Becky from Colorado

I'm a much happier person when I feel like I'm in control of my life and have a hand in shaping my future. The out-of-control spiral that was my life has stopped since I had my surgery. Such a relief!

Q: If I go ahead and have weight-loss surgery, will I be able to eat normally again?

3FC: For the first few days after your surgery, you won't be able to eat at all. You'll suck on ice chips, and drink water, protein drinks, broth, or teas, about an ounce at a time. This will gradually lead to soft foods, like baby food, cottage cheese, yogurts, and pureed foods. You will have to introduce food into your system slowly and carefully. Remember, after surgery, your holding tank will only be about the size of an egg, and overeating could be damaging, or even fatal.

Food selection depends largely on the individual, although everything that you eat should be quality food that's nutrient-rich, because you don't have very much space to satisfy your nutritional needs. Many people experience discomfort after eating sugar or fatty foods, while others seem to tolerate them well. Amy has no problems with sugar, but greasy foods cause her to "dump." Dumping has various symptoms for different people, but Amy experiences chest cramps and nausea, followed by a deep, uncontrollable sleep. The pains can be intense and scary, because chest pain is also a symptom of heart disease. It can feel like you're having a heart attack, when it's only a cramp.

So hopefully, with the help of your doctor, you will redefine what eating normally is, and you won't go back to those extra helpings of the sweet potato soufflé. Regardless of which weight-loss option you choose, surgically or otherwise, if you want to lose weight and keep it off, you must change your perception of what eating normally is and make better choices for the rest of your life.

To Market, to Market

In the first few weeks following weight-loss surgery, you may feel some emotional turmoil or even find yourself in mourning for the foods you can no longer eat. Also, considering you are recovering from surgery, it isn't a bad idea to stock the refrigerator with foods you'll be eating until you are mentally and physically up to grocery shopping again. Here's a list from Maureen from New York City, who had RGB surgery in August 2004 and since then has lost more than 130 pounds. Maureen compiled this shopping list based on what she learned from her nutritionist. The items cover the first three phases (several weeks) of postsurgical eating. Your nutritionist should give you a similar list before you have your procedure, based on your needs and the type of surgery you've had.

- Protein powders
- Broth and teas
- Smooth soups (use a blender)
- Low-sugar/low-carb yogurts
- Baby food
- Crystal Light
- Unsweetened applesauce
- Instant oatmeal, plain—no sugar added
- Whipped cottage cheese or ricotta cheese

- Soft tofu
- Fat-free or 2 percent soft American cheese slices
- Sugar-free gelatin and sugar-free pudding
- Chewable vitamins and sublingual B-12 tablets
- TUMS and chewable calcium pills

Some equipment and supplies you may find handy are a blender, a food processor, one-ounce cups (you can find these at a restaurant or wholesale supply store), and an egg poacher.

Q: I want to get weight-loss surgery, but I've read stories about people being hungry and gaining their weight back. Can you gain all your weight back after surgery?

3FC: The answer is yes, you can gain the weight back, but you won't if you follow your doctor's orders. Most failures are caused by lack of support, or the patient's lack of knowledge about how to deal with her new lifestyle. So let us tell you again: *you must eat as prescribed.*

At first, when you're on liquids only, you will be drinking your meals for nutrition more than out of hunger; most patients don't feel hungry at all after surgery. As you progress, you will begin to eat more regular food, at more regular intervals. It is up to you to stick with the eating schedule exactly as prescribed for you, no matter how quickly you are losing weight. This rapid weight loss at the beginning, called "the honeymoon period" by many of our radical chicks, happens almost effortlessly. Soon after, though, you will be relying more on your own resources as your weight decreases and your body doesn't need as many calories to survive. If you start with exercising and meal plans from the beginning, you will find it easier to stick with when it counts—in the long run.

Some of our chicks found that they were more emotionally impacted by this surgery than they could have imagined. Amy felt this way. She was not prepared for the grief she would experience when she found that her old deep-fried and whip-creamed coping mechanisms had suddenly vanished. Stress eating was her only way to deal with life's problems, and surgery doesn't change that! Long-term support and therapy are vital to getting and keeping the weight off. The surgery is a tool, and you should become skilled in its use.

Q: Will I lose all of my excess weight? I was a size 6 when I got married, but now I'm a 24. Can I get back down to my 6s?

3FC: Anything is possible, but that doesn't mean it is likely. Your body is different now from when you got married, and you may never be that small again. You will probably carry the bulk of excess skin after you lose the excess fat. You should definitely exercise and focus on strength training as soon as your doctor gives you the go-ahead, so you will be as fit as possible when you reach your goal. Instead of reaching for a size-based goal, aim for a health-based goal, and proceed from there. Keep your concerns focused more on your inside than on your outside. Of course we all want to look good, feel confident, and be happy with ourselves, but a considerable amount of patience, as well as realism, is required.

We can't predict your dress size, but we can share with you what we learned from Dr. Lockett about what *not* to do after weight-loss surgery:

- Don't alter your post-op instructions and diet.
- Don't lie around the house. Get up, get dressed, and go do things even in the early post-op period. Those who get going the fastest do the best.
- Don't weigh yourself more than once a week. Scale watchers drive themselves crazy. The goal is not to lose weight so much as to improve the medical problems associated with the weight.
- Realistic expectations are a must. Don't expect to go from 350 pounds to 120 pounds. It doesn't work that way despite what many people think.
- Don't compare your weight loss with others'.

heavy hens give it up

We all have reasons why we want to lose weight, but when you've got a lot of weight to lose, there are some unique feelings that we heavy hens alone can relate to. The comments that follow were obtained through our survey, and they are very candid. These sometimes painful, sometimes joyful thoughts reflect the special problems women face when they have over a hundred pounds to lose; they touch on the deeply emotional aspects of obesity. If you also need to lose as much as we heavy hens did, perhaps these personal thoughts will remind you that you're not alone, and help get you started on your journey toward greater health and happiness.

What We Look Forward To

- No more friction bumps on our inner thighs from walking
- Buying underwear from Victoria's Secret
- Fitting into one size fits all
- Choosing hairstyles for reasons other than camouflaging our neck
- No more reliance upon clever camera angles
- Fitting in all of the amusement park rides without fear
- No more permanent red rings around our waist
- Smiling at the security television, instead of avoiding it
- Sex without fear of hurting our mate
- Wrapping a regular-sized towel around ourselves
- Knowing the paper gown at the gynecologist will actually fit
- Choosing our bathing suit, instead of the bathing suit choosing us

• *Continued on next page* •

- Washing dishes without getting our stomachs wet
- Not wondering why people are laughing
- No more fear of plastic chairs

What We Hate About Being Overweight

- Jeans with elastic waists
- Legs too fat for dainty sandals with heels
- Wearing a T-shirt over a bathing suit
- Not tucking in shirts
- Plus size signs over the clothing racks
- More expensive clothes
- "Queen size" pantyhose
- Granny panties

Q: Will I be able to eat in restaurants after weight-loss surgery? I travel a lot, and many of my meals are on the road. I don't really want to ask the servers for advice. It's rather embarrassing.

3FC: You will be able to eat in restaurants, but you'll have to make some adjustments. One of the most difficult problems is how to deal with the portion sizes. Restaurants serve large portions, and you'll only be eating a fraction of them. Expect questions from concerned servers or managers if you are only picking at your plate. Some people don't like to announce that they have had WLS, but in some cases, you might be more comfortable just telling them and getting it out of the way, rather than assuring everybody that yes, your dinner tastes fine.

Some patients get an identification card from their surgeon, explaining that they have had WLS, so they can get permission to order from the child's menu. Ask your doctor or nutritionist if she can make something similar for you to use. Restaurants are not obligated to accommodate you, but many will. Cafeterias are great choices for WLS patients, because you can look at everything in front of you and buy only what you can eat.

If you do order straight from the menu, you can pick something from the appetizer menu or choose a couple of side orders. Be careful with the appetizer menu: many of the choices are fried, sugary, or otherwise unsuitable. If all else fails, be sure to ask for a doggy bag, and you can have leftovers two or three times!

Jiffypop's tips for successful weight loss through weight-loss surgery

Jane F. Perrotta, known as Jiffypop on 3FC, is the moderator of the Weight-Loss Surgery (WLS) forum. Once topping the scales at over five hundred pounds, and now maintaining a loss of almost three hundred pounds, she is the poster chick for successful weight-loss surgery. These are her best tips for having a successful weight loss, based on what she has learned through her own experience and through coaching others through the same process.

1. Research everything beforehand, learn all you can about the procedure, and join support groups to learn how it affects their lives.
2. Ask questions: of your primary care doctor, your surgeon, and other WLS patients. Go back and ask more questions. This is not the right choice for everyone, and no matter what you decide, someone will disagree. Once you've made your decision, ignore the naysayers.

● *Continued on next page* ●

3. Keep your eyes on the prize. Maintenance is even more important than losing. Put even more effort into maintenance than you put into navigating the presurgery evaluation and approval cycle.

4. Move yourself up in your list of priorities. The stakes are much higher after surgery than before, so make sure you have appropriate food, take your vitamins, get your blood checked regularly, and incorporate resistance training to help the calcium stay in your bones.

5. Any work you do to control your food demons *before* surgery will help you afterwards.

6. Find, and keep, a live support group, no matter how successful you feel after surgery. If your surgical group needs to make room for new patients, you may find yourself looking elsewhere to meet your needs. Look into a private group or Overeaters Anonymous, or seek a therapist who specializes in eating disorders. If you don't click with your therapist, find another one who "gets it."

7. Be prepared for changes in your relationships. Your life will change, and not everyone in your life may be willing or able to keep up.

8. Surgery won't change your emotional issues. It will help with the weight loss but not with whatever stresses or issues you may have. In fact, you will no longer be able to "eat your emotions," which can make coping more difficult until you learn new methods to handle stress.

9. Figure out how to deal with head hunger, and prepare for some degree of mourning. Get therapy or find alternate outlets to battle emotional or stress eating. (I knit!)

10. The first three months are hard. Expect a much more regimented life as you move through a staged diet, from protein shakes and liquids up to real food. It can be rocky, but it won't last. You can survive anything for three months.

11. Put your energy into figuring out how to live with the surgery rather than into trying to outsmart it. One group loses and maintains and the other group doesn't.

12. People lose at different rates, and some people, despite their best efforts, will not make their goal. Make sure you're following the rules and then stop obsessing.

13. Make the most of your honeymoon phase. Exercising and eating right will give you the best weight loss possible and will carry you throughout maintenance.

14. Your success is up to you and you alone. Including others in your plans is entirely your choice, but be aware that the fast, massive weight loss will make even the most well-meaning people wonder all kinds of bizarre things. You might have to say something if only to stop rumors that you've become a drug addict or you're dying of cancer.

15. Attitude is everything. If you go into this process thinking you're a failure or that this is a punishment for mistakes you've made in your life, you'll be miserable and have a very high risk of failure. If you embrace this as a second chance, you'll do much better.

16. Ask for help. It's out there. Even if you are bedridden or in a wheelchair, or have no cartilage in your knees, there *are* exercises you can do.

17. Realize that this is no quick fix and that you will still have to do the same hard work to get it all off and keep it off. You will need to exercise and watch what you eat for the rest of your life, just like everyone else does. Congratulations. You are normal.

Q: I am a stress eater. How will I do it with weight-loss surgery? Will I be "comforted" with smaller bites of food instead of the larger amounts I eat now?

3FC: If you are a stress eater, the first thing you must do is find another outlet for your stress. You cannot stress-eat after weight-loss surgery. It is imperative that you work on this before your procedure. You'll need to pick up a hobby, or maybe some alternate activity, like exercise or even meditation.

Amy was a classic stress eater. This was one reason we all worried about her when she had surgery. What would Amy do when things got stressful? What would she do when she was bored or lonely or anxious? We were afraid she would continue to eat, and die.

Amy has done well with portion control, and she has not suffered ill effects from stress eating, although she does still do it on occasion, but to a small degree. Amy did not realize how similar her emotional eating patterns would be after surgery. She knew her surgery would change her stomach, but it didn't occur to her that it wouldn't change her emotional response to life. Not only were life's problems and stresses still there, but she had new problems. She was afraid to swallow some foods. She was afraid of choking, or of dying. Not only was she unable to eat a lot, but she couldn't eat the same comfort foods she had in the past, like candy bars and chips. For years, food was everything for Amy. It is like that for many overweight people, so be sure that you get counseling before surgery to deal effectively with your demons.

What is the best preparation? "There may be no way to adequately prepare anyone," says Dr. Lockett. "Everyone is different and responds differently. The psychological exam that is required prior to surgery is of some value, but support groups pre- and post-op are the most important thing. All WLS patients should be in a support group, even if it is just on-line at Obesityhelp.com, for instance."

Support groups are vital for at least two years after surgery, but Amy and some other chicks at 3FC think they may prefer to stay in them for life.

The Real Skinny on Cosmetic Surgery

Tummy Tucks and Excess Skin

Excess skin is a common problem among women who have lost large amounts of weight. How much excess skin will you have? This can vary widely from one person to the next and can be affected by factors including heredity, skin tone, and time spent in the sun. Younger women will usually have less than older women, because they have more elasticity in their skin. The amount of weight you lose will also come into play, since an extra 250 pounds will have done more damage than an extra 100. How quickly you lose the weight is also important. If you lose 100 pounds fast, you stand to have more excess skin because your body didn't have time to adapt. Weight-loss surgery patients frequently face this dilemma, though it can happen to anyone. It's really impossible to know how much excess skin you will have until you get there. But carrying around the excess skin is still much better than being very overweight.

Can you prevent it? Remove it later? Our chicks have asked about this many times.

Meg Heinz, a personal trainer and one of our forum moderators, has become an expert on loose skin. After losing 120 pounds through diet and exercise, she had a considerable amount of excess skin. She researched the topic and chose to have her loose skin surgically removed. She has shared her knowledge and experience with the rest of us.

Q: Will exercise affect the way my skin looks when I reach my goal weight?

Meg: Exercise alone can't make your skin tighten up; however, building muscle as you lose weight and afterwards can help to fill up some of the loose skin.

Q: Are there any creams or lotions that I can rub on my skin that will make it tighten up?

Meg: No.

Q: Are there any vitamins or supplements that I can take that will make my skin tighten up?

Meg: No.

Q: When will I be able to tell whether my skin will tighten up after weight loss?

Meg: Try not to worry prematurely about potential skin problems before you reach your goal weight. Many body changes happen as you lose the last ten or twenty pounds. Most plastic surgeons tell you to wait at least six months after you reach your goal weight and stabilize there to see how your skin reacts to your weight loss. However, not much is likely to change after a year.

Q: I've reached my goal weight and waited six months and still have a problem with excess skin. What can I do?

Meg: At this point, it comes down to two choices: live with the skin or have it surgically removed. Excess skin problems can usually be camouflaged under clothing quite nicely. If you don't want to live with the skin, you can schedule a consultation with a plastic surgeon to discuss surgical options. You might want to consider talking to a doctor just to find out what all your options are, even if you don't think that you would consider surgery.

Q: What kinds of plastic surgeries are done for excess skin?

Meg: Here are the names of some of the various procedures:

- Arms: brachioplasty
- Thighs: thigh lift or lower body lift

- Face/neck: face lift
- Breasts: breast lift, mastopexy
- Butt: butt lift, lower body lift
- Entire lower body (abdomen, butt, thighs): lower bodylift, belt lipectomy

Many of the above can be combined with lipo to remove excess fat. Frequently multiple procedures are done together to save on expenses.

Q: Does plastic surgery leave scars?

Meg: Yes. Unfortunately it's a trade-off between scars and excess skin. Most scars can be camouflaged by clothing or a bathing suit or underwear, although those on the arms and knees and other exposed areas are more visible. Scars go through a maturation process as they heal, starting off as red and raised, and fading to thin white lines over the course of a year. Your doctor will suggest products and techniques (like massage) to minimize scarring. You need to avoid tanning and sun exposure on your scars for a year.

Q: How much does all this excess skin weigh? Will I lose weight if I get rid of the skin?

Meg: "Dry skin" (skin drained of all its fluids) doesn't weigh much at all. (They drain the fluids back into your body in the OR before they remove the skin.) Frequently, however, some fat is removed along with excess skin and that adds some weight to what's removed. The total weight can range from just a pound or two to twenty or more pounds, depending on the amount of excess skin and attached fat that you have. Everyone's experience will be different. A plastic surgeon who examines you can answer that question for you.

You can read our latest info on excess skin at www.3fatchicks.com/cosmeticsurgery.

Liposuction

If your problem is a stubborn fat deposit that you can't get rid of, liposuction might be for you. Some chicks have done all they can to master their thighs and crunch their abs, but they still have a couple of speed bumps on their curves. If this sounds like you, liposuction might be just what you need. In liposuction, a surgeon vacuums out your excess fat cells from under your skin. The surgeon will insert a hollow tube into the fatty area, basically plunge the fat loose, and suck it out. Common side effects are bruising and swelling, but as with any procedure, rare complications can occur, including death.

Lipo won't tighten up loose skin, and it won't get rid of cellulite. It will get rid of stubborn fat that just doesn't want to go away. This procedure is not intended as a method of weight loss. Even the most diligent dieter and strength trainer can be left with fat deposits that just won't budge. Lipo is, in fact, the only way you can spot-reduce. The procedure, which can be done under local anesthesia, is generally much more cost-effective than traditional cosmetic surgery. Ask your cosmetic surgeon or dermatologist if lipo can help you.

Words to Live By

All our dreams can come true, if we have the courage to pursue them.
—WALT DISNEY

In two decades I've lost a total of 789 pounds. I should be hanging from a charm bracelet. —ERMA BOMBECK

laying the golden egg

As is true of any great journey, on the road to better health and wellness, just when you think you've arrived, you realize that you are just beginning! The most important challenge in any commitment to a fitter and thinner lifestyle comes when you've already lost the weight. Keeping the weight off can take just as much effort as losing it in the first place. You can never go back to your old style of eating or eat like your thin friends, or you will regain the weight, and for good reason. You may be surprised to learn that your metabolism is slower now than it was when you were overweight or when you were originally thin. Now, perhaps more than ever, you have to really pay attention to what you are doing.

Learning how to maintain your commitment to a new lifestyle, not only during the initial weight-loss phase but for the rest of your life, is a process of getting to know yourself, emotionally and psychologically as well as physically. Many chicks gain weight through emotional eating to soothe other problems such as stress, loneliness, or troubled relationships. Maybe you were bored, or frustrated with a job that didn't challenge you. Whatever the reasons were behind your extra weight, keeping the weight off means facing those demons, and finding a better way to cope with your feelings, as well as your waistline.

We know that if you've gotten to this point, you feel much better than you did. You're more energetic, you look fabulous, and your health has improved tremendously. You have to keep this success in mind and remember what you're working for. If you back off, or let those nasty demons rear their ugly heads, it can all slip through your fingers like a greasy french fry.

We 3 fat chicks were once notorious yo-yo dieters. If our jeans were too tight, we'd follow a quick weight-loss scheme, then go back to our old eating habits. And of course, it should be no surprise that the weight came back on as quickly as it left us—and straight back onto our thighs—until we realized that we had to make a plan not just for next week or next month but also for the rest of our lives.

Losing the weight is the adventurous, exciting part of the journey. It's keeping the weight off that requires elbow grease. Our most inspirational weight loss role models have taught us a few lessons. The first lesson we learned about keeping the weight off was to actively invest in our weight maintenance on a daily basis. You can't just lose the weight and forget about it. We had already learned the little things that make a big difference in the long haul, and we couldn't forget them now. For example, we learned that if we start out the morning with exercise, we are less likely to give in to temptations later in the day. Likewise, if we take the time to measure ourselves with a tape and weigh regularly, it is easier to stay at goal, since we are aware of the slightest change in the wrong direction.

We began to understand what it meant to be fully accountable for our actions. If we screwed up, we had no one to blame but ourselves. For us, the most important difference between then and now is our commitment to ourselves, to each other, and to the support of the community of chicks that we connected with through our Web site.

The inspiration and determination to get started on the climb of your life is the first step in any successful dieting program. The next step is learning how to maintain your commitment to your new lifestyle, not only during the initial weight-loss phase but for the rest of your life. So for all of you who are trying to lay a golden egg, here are some tips from our high-maintenance chicks, to help you along on your new path, so that the next diet you go on will be your last.

The Six Golden Gateways to Successful Maintenance

1. Make Yourself a Priority

You're never going to achieve your goals as long as you're the last person on your list each day. You're going to have to give up a few things in exchange for other activities if you want to keep off this weight. You may think that your life is too busy to accommodate your new lifestyle, but it isn't. You simply can't keep putting yourself at the end of the schedule. Diet and exercise are a priority for health, just like practicing good hygiene or visiting a doctor when you're sick. You're not selfish for putting your health ahead of washing your husband's underwear! When you take care of your health, you benefit your whole family. Beverly learned this and, as a result, has lost 190 pounds. By making herself a priority in her own life, she has kept the weight off.

Beverly from Arkansas

I absolutely have to make taking care of myself a priority or I would never bother. I could come up with a hundred excuses for putting off exercise, like eating crap out of convenience and pretending the dryer is shrinking my clothes. But where would that get me? Oh yeah, I remember, my old life! We have to take care of ourselves in order to be the best possible wives, moms, and women we can be, period. Do I feel guilty sometimes? Absolutely! But I figure I can still take my daughter to the park an hour from now, after I exercise. The laundry will get done . . . eventually; the floor doesn't need to be vacuumed right this minute. It's a trade-off—learning how to balance all the most important things in life to achieve the best possible outcome. So, everybody is not completely happy all of the time? They will get over it. Plus—and you all know it's true—if momma ain't happy, ain't nobody happy!

maintenance mantras

Many of our high-maintenance chicks have mantras that they describe as the little voice in their head that spurs them on when they feel like giving up. We asked them to share some of these inspirational "hooks" with us, so that you can try out a few for yourself. Repeat some of these maintenance mantras to yourself the next time you need a pep talk!

Falling down is not failure. Failure is staying down.
— MEL, PERSONAL TRAINER, MODERATOR OF 3FC

It gets easier over time . . . It gets easier over time . . .
— JENNIFER, NEW YORK

Never trade what you want at the moment for what you want the most.
— BEVERLY, ARKANSAS

You can quit this very second if you really want, but is that what you really want to do? — JAN, FLORIDA

Is——(fill in the blank with your favorite forbidden food) really worth sixty minutes of cardio? — MELANIE, MODERATOR OF 3FC

I don't do that anymore. — MEG, MODERATOR OF 3FC

Breathe: it can change the pattern of your thoughts. Learn to wait: once you can wait, you can do almost anything. And remember: it all counts. — ROBIN, CALIFORNIA

hazard signs on the hungry highway

One of the most difficult parts of maintaining weight loss is that we fat chicks, like most of the rest of the world, have an epic capacity for denial. We can feel like we're steering clear of temptation and never even notice that the road we're on is headed straight to the nearest burger stand. So for all of us queens of denial, who can wind up ten pounds heavier faster than you can say chocolate chip cheesecake, here's a few of the hazard signs and suggestions for how to steer out of your skid.

Danger Signs

- I forget to eat a snack and then I'm so hungry that I overeat at mealtime.
- I do not want to exercise, and I start making excuses to myself.
- I start picking leftovers off my kids' plates.
- I stop drinking water, which only makes things worse.
- I start picking and nibbling at high-calorie food—a slippery slope that leads right to a binge.
- I buy or make certain food for "others." Who am I kidding? It's really for me and I'm the one who ends up eating it.
- I don't have food planned or prepared in advance. And I sure don't make very good decisions when I'm hungry!

How to Steer Out of Your Skid

- I carry fruit and veggies for snacks everywhere I go.
- I try to exercise more.
- I stop buying treats "for the kids."
- I try to be accountable for what I eat.

• *Continued on next page* •

- I try to pay more attention to my positive inner voice, and I say my mantras a lot.
- I steer clear of trigger items.
- I pay more attention to water consumption.
- I plan ahead, so nothing is left to chance.
- I try to get more rest.

2. It's Okay to Slip Up a Little

A successful diet is not an all-or-nothing approach. That would be a miserable, not to mention impossible, way to diet! To err is human, so don't expect yourself to be perfect. Slipping up doesn't have to mean you'll gain the weight back, though. Just accept that you cheated a little, and then move on and try to stay on program the next time you're tempted. How many times have you said, "I've already blown my diet today, I may as well keep eating and start my diet again tomorrow"? The second you realize you've goofed up, just stop. Don't wait until tomorrow, because you're guaranteed to feel worse then. If you stop now, you can feel proud of yourself later, knowing that you realized what was happening and you took control.

One thing you do have to keep in mind, though, is that you can't have continual slip-ups. If you are constantly experiencing setbacks, then you should reevaluate your lifestyle, because you will put the weight back on if you keep it up. When you chose your weight-loss diet, we hope you picked a diet plan you could stick with, because you usually have to keep it up for the rest of your life. It becomes a lifestyle, not a diet. You eat just a little more than you did while losing weight. You keep up the exercise and continue to make good choices. You can have slipups or even planned treats, but you need to draw the line at what defines success and maintenance. Decide how far you can go without losing control, and whatever you do, don't cross that line.

Jamie found a realistic diet plan that she could live with for the rest of her life, and in her case, the right diet has made all the difference to her long-term weight-loss success.

Jamie from North Carolina

I can't count how many times I reached my goal weight and then gained the pounds right back. I never really ate bad foods, I just ate too much food. I was fooling myself to think I could go on a strict diet that I usually hated, one where I couldn't wait to get back to "normal" food, which I usually overate. Enough was enough. The last time I decided to lose weight, I wanted to eat my regular foods, since I knew I'd get back there eventually. So I counted every calorie that passed through my lips, and I exercised, since it was all about calories in versus calories out. I couldn't believe how much easier this was for me! When I reached goal, I kept on counting calories and just ate a little more. I still exercise, since it's also part of the big picture. I learned the hard way that I couldn't avoid paying attention, just because I was at goal. If you don't keep track of what you are eating and doing, the weight will slip back on before you know it. Good health should last forever, but it only happens if you make it happen.

3. Long-Term Success Isn't Automatic

Some things in life simply don't come without some hard work up front. We would much rather have the weight loss occur instantly and never have to worry about gaining it back, but it won't happen that way. Weight loss requires patience and hard, consistent work. In the world of weight-loss maintenance, there is no immediate gratification, and no buy-now, pay-later plans. You have to put your cash on the barrel every time you eat a meal. Here's how one of our most successful high-maintenance chicks explains it:

Barb from Ontario

I think that as a society, we are conditioned to live on credit. Buy a house, live in it now, and pay for the next twenty-five years. Buy a car, drive it now, and pay for it the next five years. Weight loss is not like that. You can't decide to lose weight and get fit and be a size 8 in good shape today

*and then pay later. You have to work now for results later, which is not
something we're all used to doing anymore!*

*So why do some people start losing, keep losing, and then maintain
their weight loss while others fail? I think it is mostly a mind-over-matter
thing with a lot of determination thrown in. I recently realized that it was
like a snowball rolling downhill. We only have to summon the determination to start the thing rolling in the first place, and then it will gain momentum on its own. Success causes more effort and effort causes more
success. Then we just have to find it within ourselves to give it the occasional push when it starts to slow or stall. I think that's where most people
fail. The momentum stops and they are resigned to let it.*

4. Move It or Lose It

The chances are slim to none that you will achieve your weight-loss
goal without exercise, and you have even less of a chance at keeping
that weight off without it. Exercise is not only a calorie burner; it is essential to our system. Our hearts and lungs and bones need a solid
cardio and strength-training program. The members of our Maintain-
ers' Forum unanimously agree that exercise is part of a weight-loss
maintenance success.

Anne from Arizona

*Exercise is just fantastic! Possibly the best thing I've done for myself. I went
from total couch potato to triathlete, and no, I didn't even have to get a perfect body to make that happen. I feel so much better, so much more relaxed,
and so much more in control when I exercise. I'm still exercising now that
I'm pregnant, but I've dropped the frequency, intensity, and duration quite
a bit. Once you get started exercising, it is so tough to quit. Even when I
broke my foot last year, I still managed to go swimming and pool running
with a floaty belt. There is always a way, no matter what's going on in your
life, to fit in a little healthy activity!*

5. Forget the Head Games

Emotional eating can slow down or destroy our attempts at weight loss
and maintenance. Eating is not always about the food; often it's about

how food makes us feel. It can be comforting or distracting, or give us a sense of pleasure we don't always get elsewhere. Although this kind of emotional eating comforts us in the moment, we always feel lousy afterward. Guilt, shame, physical discomfort—these are just some of the aftereffects of emotional eating. And we *know* we're going to regret it later, but we still do it anyway. Now is the time to get over it. Learn some new habits. We lost our weight, not our problems, so it's important to deal with your issues and find a better solution than eating. Plan ahead, so you have some recourse the next time an emotional food craving hits.

Mette from Norway

I've always known that I overeat when I'm very hungry. I also overeat when I feel depressed, rejected, sad, and down. I do tend to take care of myself with sweets: eating cookies always makes me feel better!

The changes in my routine felt stressful because I didn't want to make them—like exchanging cookies for dumbbells! Feeling anxious and insecure didn't help either. I even managed to identify new high-risk situations for overeating: I noticed that I also overeat when I don't sleep enough, drink enough water, or rest when I'm tired. It's weird that I interpret every signal of discomfort from my body as a sign to eat, but I found a way to turn to exercise and real self-love—rather than just consuming mass quantities of empty calories—and that, in the long run, was truly a comfort!

fat fiction

All chicks need a curvy heroine! Read a few of these books recommended by some of our chicks for another perspective

• Continued on next page •

on being overweight. From chubby girls to scorned women, you'll find stories to make you laugh and cry and hopefully become inspired in your own weight loss. You can see a current list of all of the favorites at www.3fatchicks.com/books.

Blubber, Judy Blume
Bridget Jones's Diary, Helen Fielding
Fat Chance, Deborah Blumenthal
Good in Bed, Jennifer Weiner
In Her Shoes, Jennifer Weiner
Lady Oracle, Margaret Atwood
Life in the Fat Lane, Cherie Bennett
Losing It, Lindsay Faith Rech
Night Swimming, Robin Schwarz
One Fat Summer, Robert Lipsyte
Slim Chance, Jackie Rose
Something's Wrong with Your Scale, Van Whitfield
What Are You Looking At? The First Fat Fiction Anthology, Donna
　Jarrell, Ira Sukrungruang

6. Lifelong Success Is Not Just Wishful Thinking

In a nation where everyone is dieting but obesity rates continue to rise, it seems like weight-loss success is just wishful thinking, but it's not. Lifelong success is completely within our reach, but you have to make a conscious effort to make it happen. We're not going to kid you; it will be hard work. You'll have to work at it for the rest of your life. The good news is that it does become a lot easier after a while, and you'll soon learn that you don't want to do it any differently.

Meg from Pennsylvania
Three years of living maintenance every day has given me the confidence of knowing that the only way that I'll gain the weight back is if I make a lot of

really bad choices. I now know—beyond the shadow of a doubt—that the power to keep the weight off is totally in my hands.

Regaining isn't going to happen to me passively; I would actively and consciously have to make bad decisions—ranging from not monitoring my weight to not exercising to eating the wrong foods—in order to put the weight back on. Knowing that keeping the weight off is completely under my control and in my hands makes maintenance a lot easier in my mind. I know what to do to keep the weight off and I fully intend to keep doing it every day of my life. This new body (and new life) is a gift beyond compare, and I'll never ever choose to give it up.

Last Words That We Hope Will Last a Lifetime

There are no quick fixes to lifelong problems, and dieting is no exception. When we make a decision to diet, we are making a decision to change our life, and everything we do from that point forward, no matter how small or how grand, will impact our success. Our hope is that you will take the knowledge and experience that we've offered you in these pages and put them to use for the rest of your life, because the diet never really ends, it just becomes a better lifestyle. And if you take nothing else away with you, we, and all of the chicks who have contributed to this book, hope you realize that no matter how tough the struggle may seem at times, you are not alone!